The
LOVE
Inside Me

İÇİMDEKİ AŞK

The story of eight women from five countries in the pursuit of
their dreams of having babies....

NUR YILMAZ RUPPI

SAINT MICHAEL'S PRESS

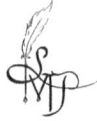

A SAINT MICHAEL'S PRESS BOOK
4 WEEMS LANE, NO 133
WINCHESTER, VA 22601

stmichaelspress.com

Cover photograph by Cosimo Ruppi
Cover design and layout by Veronica El-Showk
Executive editor: Natalie M. Hartman
Translated by Nihal Gökçe

All medical information/recommendations reviewed by Dr. Yücel Karaman,
head of Endoscopic Surgery and IVF Department at the Edith Cavell Medical
Institute and Hospital Français in Brussels, Belgium.

Original edition published in Turkish before being translated into English for
this Saint Michael's Press edition.

ISBN 978-0-9903754-6-3 (softcover)
ISBN 978-0-9903754-7-0 (electronic version)

PRINTED IN THE UNITED STATES OF AMERICA

About the Author

NUR YILMAZ RUPPI was born in Istanbul in 1970. She studied architecture at Yıldız Technical University in Istanbul. While working as an interior architect she started writing for Milliyet's weekend supplements, one of the most prominent newspapers in Turkey. She also worked as an editor at TASARIM (Design Magazine), prepared decoration pages, and wrote articles in L'Officiel. She has contributed travel essays to DISHY women's magazine as well as to Vizyon Dekorasyon magazine and Home-Art Dekorasyon magazine. She also wrote the columns titled 'Hola Barcelona' and 'Hola Avrupa' in a women's magazine called ELELE for more than five years. Today she writes for DDmag. it, an online Italian design magazine, and a Turkish-English lifestyle magazine called Hillsider. She is married with two sons and currently lives in Italy where she's a designer and writes as a freelance journalist.

This is her first book. 'The Love Inside Me' is the real life story about her journey to becoming a mother. It was originally published in Turkish before being translated into English for this edition.

For Cosimo, Matteo, and Leo

Contents

Introduction

My Passion for Writing

How did I come up with the idea of writing this book? First of all, writing is a need for me. I have always been writing in my mind if I have not actually put pen to paper. It makes me happy to narrate and share. I don't like keeping things to myself... So it all happened by itself. It became a mission for me to write this book. I'd read several books about pregnancy and birth during my pursuit of having a baby, which were theoretically satisfying, but left me emotionally unsatisfied. I had always heard second-hand stories of other women like me who had trouble having children. Those were our stories and we were the ones who had to tell them. This made me feel I needed to write this book.

I am an architect by profession and not a writer, but I have been writing ever since I learned to read and write. My passion for writing first started with diaries, followed by correspondence with my friends in other cities, bringing depth and excitement to my life. I belong to a generation who gets excited when opening the mailbox in the morning. In an era where we had to go through an operator to place a phone call and we didn't know the first thing about computers, we used to put pen to carefully selected paper to transport our feelings. Our letters would travel hundreds of miles before reaching their recipient in days. It felt normal for us. It was the way it was. We couldn't imagine otherwise; we communicated by mail; we wrote a lot of letters; we wrote more than we spoke; we wrote as if we were speaking... In secondary school, two close friends of mine and I issued a school magazine. Young as we were, we used to interview the actors and actresses of the City Theaters who visited our tiny town of Tekirdağ monthly, for the magazine, which developed our self-confidence naturally. My passion for writing took me from the school magazine to newspapers to decoration and fashion magazines and I kept pursuing it nonstop. It had gotten under my skin. I set off to write this book with the support of the lovely people around me who kept telling me I should definitely write a book. And, I wanted to share my experiences, both happy and sad, so that other women like me would read them and feel they were not alone.

As Paulo Coelho said, "I write to understand my soul."

I couldn't have put it better myself.

How Did I Write This Book?

I wrote this book in maybe a hundred different places in over ten cities. I started in Brussels; I went on in Tekirdağ and Istanbul. I revised it in Treviso and Udine, in Italy. In the meantime, I took short trips to Venice, Naples, Florence, Bari, Gökçeada, Bozcaada, Marmara Island, and Bodrum... Each town, with its sights, smells, and ambiance stirred different inspirations, and I kept on writing. And, I finally wrote the last line in Vicenza. My little white laptop named 'Eee' went everywhere with me. At home it usually sat on my desk, but sometimes on the dinner table, the kitchen counter, or my bed. It strolled with me from parks to cafés, from tea gardens to restaurants. I took it to the mall and to the gym, held it on my lap, sitting on a wall by the street, in a van, on the train, in the subway, in the car, on the plane—basically everywhere I had the opportunity I kept writing. This book was not written page by page, but literally sentence by sentence. After all, the book can wait, but babies cannot. There were times where I was so busy taking care of my sons that I had to neglect my writing. Some days I only wrote a single sentence, some days I didn't even touch the keyboard. But my passion for writing and my mission kept me going. I managed to finish my book in two years, every day of which was very enjoyable, but not always easy.

First Thoughts...

Baby or Career?

We read interviews in newspapers where celebrities are asked whether they plan on having children. The answer is usually that they do but keep postponing it. Not this summer, not this winter, not yet, not before this project is over, let's first deal with this, let's move to a new house first... Our families are tired of asking us, they've given up. We might surprise them sometime, but we really don't know when. Sometime, when we have the time...

Having a Baby = Lower Pay

An article in an Italian newspaper reported the results of a survey about women. The statistics were striking: The duration of time women are kept away from work on account of family reasons is 14.7 years on average, where it is merely 1.6 years for men. Women do two thirds of all the work worldwide to make only ten percent of the total income. They own only one percent of all the land and make up 70 percent of the population of 1.2 billion living in poverty.

Multitasking women, women who don't know how to keep

up with what they are expected to do, women who can deal with a hundred tasks at once without complaining, women who strive selflessly to end up with nothing! So many of them struggle until the end of their lives without being able to get one square foot of land for themselves. These bitter facts may seem distant to us, yet, they are true for the women we see around us every day... Our mothers were probably the last generation of non-working women, today most women work. Not only are they more educated and now can find work more easily, but they are forced to work because a single salary is not enough to provide for a family in urban life. Therefore, the duties of women have increased. It's not enough anymore that they are in charge of the children, the house work, cooking, cleaning, shopping, and they have their duties as a wife, they now have to go to work, too! So, basically, women have to work full-time all their waking hours.

According to a study cited by Financial Times' prominent economic columnist Tim Harford, women in their 30's who delay having their first baby by one year make 10 percent more in total during their lifetime, compared to women who don't have babies. How encouraging is that for women who think about having a baby?! The article goes on to say that the cost of a career break is outrageously high. For instance, whereas the earnings and advancement of women without children are comparable to those of their male counterparts, a gap forms immediately as a child comes on the scene. The woman who has a baby will not receive any pay raise or promotion for a while even if she continues to work, and will incur a 40 percent decrease in salary if she decides to have a break. In a way she is punished for having a child. Although she has to work much harder physically and mentally both at work and at home, she is not rewarded but punished for it, not exactly fair, is it? It's almost as if we lived in China, where you are fined for having children as part of the one-child population policy.

Women who think they have a lot of time ahead of them and decide to postpone getting pregnant, believing they can always have a baby later, start facing problems conceiving as they age. There are those who are ready to have a child, but don't have the time as they work. There are those who seek to find the right partner with whom to have a child late in life. Those who have to wait because of economic reasons, even though they have been married for a long time... The list goes on. We all have our own good reasons for waiting, but the one inevitable cause is that it becomes harder to conceive today than it used to be because women go beyond the optimal age to have a baby. They say one should strike while the iron is hot, but it is not easy to know when!

The Fear of Becoming a Mother

Sometimes we may be physically ready to be a mother, but we may not feel mentally so. As the idea of a baby forms in our mind we are overwhelmed with care. It's hard to put our thoughts in order. We keep asking ourselves whether we can make it. Am I going to be a good mother? Am I going to be able to care for my baby's needs? Am I going to have to give up my work? Am I going to miss having a career? How is it going to affect my relationship with my partner? Am I ever going to be able to go back to my old life, to spend time with my friends? Am I going to change – physically and mentally – after I have children? Where women in their forties who want to grab their chance of having a baby are concerned, other worries add to these. That is, there are so many risks involved with getting pregnant after 40. Expectant mothers experience drastic changes in their body. Young women's bodies are able to tolerate and adapt to these changes easily whereas women who conceive after 40 struggle with cardiovascular, respiratory, renal, genital, bone, breast, skin and especially womb problems. For instance, the amount of blood in our body increases by 50 %, adding to the heart's load. If the expectant mother has no health problems and has good organ reserve, she doesn't experience problems. If, however, there are any health conditions, pregnancy aggravates them. As we get heavier our problems do, too. Conditions such as diabetes or hypertension worsen; preeclampsia and cardiovascular problems are encountered more frequently. So, in addition to the fear of becoming a new mother, there is also the fear of being an older mother...

An Act of Courage...

There are things in life which you keep dreaming of but never gather the courage to accomplish. They may be trivial, but we somehow magnify them in our mind. Qualms, concerns, lack of confidence, genetic codes, environmental factors, or family pressure stand between us and our longings. We feel our life would change and we would lose control if we ever tried and realized our dreams. Change is scary while it doesn't cost a thing to dream.

We, humans, dream of innumerable things and add new ones to the list every day. But then one day we want to be a mother. This is the best of all the dreams we've ever had, but maybe also the hardest to make true because it involves a radical decision, with no going back. This is going to be our greatest responsibility in life; we are going to be responsible for a person for our whole life, unlike a job that we might quit when we've had enough. But then, when a woman wants to have a baby, she accepts all this. Even though conceiving and giving birth to a healthy child may look easy enough, we know it's hard and risky. This is the privilege of being a woman. Your fears and concerns just evaporate as if you weren't the one who didn't dare pursuing so many of your dreams. Everything seems insignificant except your baby. Your maternal instinct gives you incredible power. And your life will be divided into two episodes from now on: before and after pregnancy...

It Turns Out You Can't Have a Baby at the Drop of a Hat

I was 30 and my husband 38 when we got married. We both loved children. We wanted to have a baby straight away as we didn't fancy being older parents. Furthermore, we were about to leave Istanbul to go overseas and I wanted to give birth in my own country, with my family near me.

You cannot plan life. Seven years passed and we spent all seven trying to have a baby. I was pregnant a total of five times, with more doctors helping me than I can remember, in eight different hospitals, in four countries with four different languages and religions. The first three of my pregnancies ended in the loss of six babies. So many tests were run, not indicating a specific problem. When you don't have a problem, you can't find a solution. But I couldn't have a baby! I was desperate, but still hopeful. They said there was nothing wrong with me, but I was so frustrated I just couldn't feel like a normal, healthy woman. The doctors finally decided to take no further risks, and when I valiantly got pregnant for the fourth time they took every possible measure to keep the baby safe. I went through my whole pregnancy lying in bed. I was given a cervical cerclage, innumerable pills, and shots both on the belly and the buttocks. I was continuously monitored through ultrasound imaging. I observed the doctors' recommendations religiously and finally was able to hold my baby in my arms.

My fifth pregnancy came purely by chance. I had no intention of getting pregnant again when I realized I was, in fact, pregnant, which made me laugh at myself. I had been pregnant so many times, I had gathered enough knowledge about pregnancy to write a dissertation about it, and yet I had failed to notice I was pregnant right away. It was my seventh week when I found out I was expecting. For weeks I had been beating myself up for being hungry and sleepy all the time. The baby was almost two months old! The news came as an exhilarating surprise. It added new color and dimension to my book, which I embraced with more enthusiasm, for I was now going to write with different emotions as a fledgling mother and an expectant woman.

I thought what I'd been through separated me from other women, but as shared my story I came across so many that had been through the same or similar experiences... There are hundreds, thousands of women struggling to have a baby. Some of us let others in while some of us keep to ourselves. There are those who strive to find a solution and consult physician after physician to get help, and those who choose to ignore the problem or stop trying, maybe because of socio-cultural or economic issues... Those who give up their dream of having a baby and those who keep trying, hoping for the day when they will be able to hold their baby...

This book is about my efforts to be a mother... In it you will find my story in full detail and witness my multicultural adventures... You will also find the stories of other women who have risked and sacrificed a lot to have a baby. Where we are now may be a result of our choices or our fate. Maybe we planned to be parents, maybe it all came unexpectedly. Maybe, although we don't have children, there is nothing we want more, and maybe we will one day find ourselves pregnant after years of unsuccessful attempts.

Whoever we are, wherever we live, we, as women, are a combination of our many desires. Some claim that the desire to be a mother is instinctive, while some deny it... No matter what others might say or think, many of us have one common desire regardless of age, time or place: WE JUST WANT A BABY!

Finally, a Few More Words...

The fertilized egg attaches itself to the womb and a new life begins to burgeon. From a single cell it grows to being millimeters and then centimeters long. It takes life and comes into the world. All this happens in just nine months. The creation of a human being is nature's greatest miracle. Nature has already created the greatest work of art and there is no competing with it!

I was trying to conceive and I couldn't, and when I could I kept losing the baby. While I kept on trying, I wanted to read the stories of other women who had been through the same adventure, but I searched several bookstores in vain without coming across a book on this subject. So, I started to write both what I was going through and what was going on around me.

I had everything I wanted to write laid out in my mind, but it took time for it all to come together. It is by coincidence that the book started to take shape as my baby sprouted inside my body; they grew up together, but the book was born first. Just as it takes a lot of patience and perseverance to nurture and raise a baby, so it does to write a book. Thousands of words carefully collected from not only your experiences and emotions, but also those of the people around you, that come together to constitute it.

There is nothing more fulfilling than seeing your baby grow and accomplishing a task you've undertaken – especially if you feel you are doing something useful. We, women, have an instinctive desire to create, be it a human being or a work of art, a book or an object, it gives us pleasure to be productive.

What I have written is both about myself and the other women to whom I somehow connected through our common experiences. Even though we had come from different places on earth, we had a common desire; we just wanted to have a baby. We understood each other: the people, emotions, and lives who constitute this book have therefore flown into the pages spontaneously...

If you define yourself as one of these women, you may find in this book answers to your questions from different perspectives. Our experiences may overlap, even though our paths may never cross...

May you be granted all that you ever wish for...

1

Tekirdağ

The day my brother was born, November 10th, 1979, was the happiest of my life of nine and a half years. How awesome it was, the birth of a baby! I was a big sister and I now had a big responsibility for life—to protect my little brother. I held this new born baby in my arms, I inhaled his sweet scent. He was my blood, my life.

My parents, who knew I had been wishing for a brother for a long time, let me name him. I named him Can, after my mother's doctor, long before it became a popular name throughout Turkey. I liked it both because of its lovely meaning—life, soul—and because of its catchy, monosyllabic sound like my own name, Nur.

I remember my mother coming out of the labor room, tired but happy. Seeing her made me think what an incredible feeling it must be for a woman to be a mother, to bring a human being into the world. Was I going to be a mother one day?

❧

I could never forget the moment when my mother told me I was going to have a little brother. That moment 30 years ago affected me so deeply that I remember it in vivid detail. I was in third grade in elementary school and a two-shift system had been adopted that year for the first time due to the increasing number of pupils, with a morning- and an afternoon-shift; you had to be in the morning shift for one term and in the afternoon shift for the other. That term I was in the afternoon shift. One morning, the postman left an envelope at our doorstep. My mother opened it excitedly and after a quick glance at the contents turned to me to say, "You know what it says? You are going to have a little brother or sister!" I was in the clouds.

My mother tells me that I was so very caring towards young children and I enjoyed spending time with them so much that they had decided I had to have a sibling. One day, our form teacher asked me to tell my mother to come and see her. I remember being scared at first: was there something the matter with my schoolwork? Or, was it because I wanted to rush through my homework to go out to play as it was spring time?

My mother came to school to speak to our teacher the next day. Anxious, I waited outside the classroom for them to come out. Our teacher Mrs. Nural and my mother came out smiling. Mrs. Nural caressed me on the head and said, "So you are soon to be a big sister, now I can see why you are so excited."

My mother held my hand firmly and, looking at me said, "I'm sure Nur will be a wonderful big sister."

Had my lovely mother become even more beautiful during her pregnancy? Especially during the last months—my favorite thing was to stroke her taut belly, which seemed to me just about to explode. I thought I was caressing my little brother or sister. When it started to kick, I would be delighted and wait patiently for the next movement. Ultrasounds imaging and sonograms were unheard of yet. We didn't know the baby's gender, but as it kicked very hard people kept saying, "this one is a boy, he will be a footballer, too." And I believed it with all the naivety of the kids of my generation... The long awaited moment had finally arrived... And when I held my baby brother in my arms, it was the most meaningful moment of my life thus far.

❦

I had a childhood full of fun in Tekirdağ,[*] between the sea on one side and vines and orchards on the other. Among my flamboyant memories of a great childhood are the days when we visited the gipsy quarters. Those cheerful people lead a life that I contemplated with wonder. It was considered a most normal thing when the casual workers working in the fields just decided not to show up. My mother and I enjoyed accompanying my father in his rounds to the quarter to gather and bring them back to work.

The quarter was utterly different from where we lived, more colorful, livelier. After seeing the people up there everything back downtown seemed dull because the gypsies, whose motto was 'spend what you earn today, tomorrow will take care of itself,' turned each day into a holiday celebrated out in the streets with all the neighbors. In summer and winter alike, the doors of the houses were always kept open, all the houses resounded with music. You

---

[*]Tekirdağ, which used to be a city of a population of 40 to 50 thousand consisting mostly of native Tekirdağ and Thrace families, has had its share of the flow of immigrants to neighboring Istanbul and the west of Turkey. It has become popular due to the high living standards it offers, and its being in close vicinity to Istanbul with a much lower cost of living. Its population has now surpassed 150 thousand.

would often come across people who played the chalice drum and danced in the street, and the youth could be seen parading with their tape players on their shoulders. Household chores, like laundry, washing up and cooking, were done outside, together with all the neighbors, chatting and singing. And the people were always merry, clad in brightly colored clothes and glittery jewelry, looking ready to go to a wedding party. I used to ask my mother why they had so many children and why the children were always out in the street. She said they didn't mind having many children as they raised them in the street, which didn't make much sense to me. I understood what she meant only after many years, when I had kids of my own.

Years went by, I started high school. I was a hardworking student. But I was also starting to realize that I was a young lady as I had a number of fans waiting outside the school to see me. I enjoyed the attention, it boosted my confidence, but it didn't mean that much to me, school came first. We lived in a small city where everyone knew each other, dating was taboo. It would put you in the spotlight, surrounded by rumors and gossip. I had no serious relationships as a young girl, just a few summer dates. Getting married didn't even cross my mind; there was so much I had to do: I had to be an architect, to travel the world, to learn foreign languages… Marriage would tie me down.

I had known my best friend Özlem since elementary school. We were inseparable. Then we became a trio with the addition of Neslihan, and then a quartet with Aslı. We had named our small gang NÖNA, from our initials. We discovered life and ourselves together, we shared the excitement of the transition from childhood to youth, of first loves, first dates; the pressure of exams and the thrill of starting university. We were kids raised in a good family environment, we had not been deprived. We were then attending good, public, and strict high schools. We used to like to talk about the future and dream of going to go to the University in Istanbul together, becoming business women, getting married and having children and always living in the same city and remaining best friends forever. We made our dreams come true, we were accepted to university and started sharing an apartment in Istanbul.

But after a while our fondness for each other was not enough to hold us together. We realized that the real world was different from what we had dreamt it to be. While we had spent each and every day together at school and outside through junior and senior high school, now that we shared an apartment circumstances had changed. Being flat mates hadn't brought us closer but estranged us. Our circles of friends, pursuits, and social activities were separated as we went off to different universities. We started to drift apart even though we loved each other. I was the first to move out. After the second year, I went to London for summer school to learn English, where I was inspired by the young people living alone, so after coming back home I went to my father to declare I had decided to move to an apartment on my own. Although he objected at first, with time he relented and gave me his support.*

---

* Özlem graduated from medical school, married her university boyfriend Asım and moved to the USA. She still lives there with her husband, who is a doctor, like her, and their two daughters. Aslı studied tourism in the UK and upon returning home started to work for a textile company, married a German man she met at work. They have a son and live in Istanbul. Nesli, the only one of the four of us who went back to Tekirdağ, started her own pharmacy and married her boyfriend in Tekirdağ. She has a daughter,

In the university, my father used to send me to the UK every summer for language education. I always chose to go to London as I admired big city life. Those who take language courses in the UK often prefer to stay on campuses in cities like Oxford and Cambridge, but I preferred the metropolitan city of London and let myself be taken by its charm and energy. I was merely 18, but being an alien in the big city didn't scare me, but excited me. I felt myself at home in Europe...

The Italian language and culture had always fascinated me. During my childhood there was a single TV station broadcasting in Turkey, the national TV channel TRT, and one of my favorite programs was the Rafaella Carra Show. When we played pop stars, the singer we liked best to mimic was Ajda, followed by Rafaella Carra and the guests on her show. We used to wrap ourselves in the shiny scarves my grandmother had brought from her pilgrimage to Mecca, pretend the pencils we held in our hands were microphones, and sing along with the TV, years before karaoke became a sweeping trend. Even back then, people used to say I had a gift for foreign languages, I do in fact pick new languages up rather quickly, but I attribute it to practicing a lot rather than being gifted, as I'm not afraid of making mistakes and always try to talk even though I may make a mess of it, I am not ashamed of struggling, with a dictionary in my hand, I try to

---

loves living in Tekirdağ and even though she occasionally complains about it, she knows she couldn't live anywhere else.

decipher everything I see on the streets, newspapers, magazines, or on TV.

Some of my best friends at the summer school in London were Italian, which was my first real exposure to the Italian culture. In London, I had acquired a circle of friends, most of whom were Italian or British. I met Aiasha in the gym. We were both very young, but she was a married woman, whereas I was a university student who didn't even dream of getting married. I was 20 and she 26. During the last 20 years, both of our lives have seen great changes. She divorced her husband Ravi, a Sri Lankan tycoon and billionaire. She met a British accountant in Bodrum, where we had gone for a holiday together, and opted for love rather than money. She is now happy with him and they have two great kids. She has named her daughter Stazia after Simply Red's 'Stars' which they used to play a lot in Halikarnas' nightclub in Bodrum that summer of 1991.

While I studied architecture, I had joined EASA, a club of European architecture students. This allowed me to join workshops in different countries each summer. I once took part in a workshop in Sweden with four of my friends from the university. We combined the workshop with a journey through the continent. We toured all of Europe by train for a month with our rucksacks and sleeping bags. We were especially impressed by Italy. If I was told then that I was going to find the man I would marry in a country of which I didn't even speak the language, I would have laughed. Destiny was slowly bringing me closer to Italy.

I first decided to learn Italian because Italy ruled in architecture, decoration, design, and furniture and it would allow me to follow the literature. Seeing I wasn't going to be able to do it in Turkey, I grasped the first opportunity that came my way and went to Florence to stay with Elif, a childhood friend, who was studying architecture in Italy. Although my initial plan was to stay for three months, I prolonged my stay as I had fallen in love with Italy. I couldn't get enough of living there. A year flew by and I was seriously considering settling in Italy.

I went back to Turkey that summer to see my family and go to some job interviews after which I intended to return to Italy. That's when I met him, the Volcano, in Istanbul one afternoon in August. It was love at first sight... and it turned my life upside down. I did go back to Italy as I had planned but came back almost immediately. Volcano, who I believed really loved me, had followed me there to convince me that it didn't make sense for me to stay on any longer. He turned my head, changed my plans, and convinced me to go back to Turkey. He had virtually brainwashed me. He had amazing persuasion skills and way with words. As a young girl of 25 years of age, I had fallen in love with a 37 year-old, experienced man who had been married and divorced, with two grown up sons, and I had put my ambitions and my ability to judge situations too, on the back burner... temporarily.

As the main character of that stormy relationship, he was the first one who put the idea of having a child in my head. He used to say he wanted us to have a daughter who resembled me. But as I played a joke on him on April Fools' Day, I realized he was far from being sincere, and the joke I played on him was an eye opener for me. It made me reconsider the relationship I had been a part of, only half-awake, for the last two years. When he woke up that morning I took his hand and put it on my belly, and said, "Your wish for a baby girl may soon come true, you know? I have great news, I'm pregnant."

I will never forget the expression of terror I saw on his face. I hadn't planned to test him, it was just an innocent joke that I thought would cheer him up, because he had been going on about a baby girl. "Oh, no, now?" he stammered." Come on, this can't be! I am not ready for another child, I have to think of my children's future; they come first for me." He was at a loss, desperate. I decided to put an end to it and stop the joke.

An April Fools' Day joke had made me see things that I had failed to see before and reconsider my relationship. The promises he made that he wanted to build a family with me were just lies to trick me. On the other hand, he was a severely jealous man who constantly tried to keep me under control and he had mood swings. I could never have been happy with him. Trying to spend one's life with someone like that would mean to be in constant need of a therapist. I could now see the future and wanted to get away from him before I got in trouble, but it wasn't easy to do since he depended on me. He said he couldn't live if I left him. He threatened me and swore he would get even. I grew even more scared after he came to my work and made a scene and called my mother and friends to make threats about me. I had put up with this obsessive man for two years. After we broke up he kept calling me to say he had changed and he insisted to see me. I resisted and I terminated my relationship with him once and for all, I felt I had made the best decision. I went back to being my old self, after two years of oppression, I was Nur the extrovert again.

Because of the mark this relationship had left on me, I felt nauseated when I thought of the pressure of men on women and I believed that I would be happier on my own than in a relationship, that I'd never suffer for the lack of a man in my life. I couldn't say I experienced a lot of family pressure growing up. My parents did set certain limits as all parents raising girls do. Even though, as a teenager, I was often mad at them and rebelled against them, I now understand the reason behind their actions very well. My family thought me to be a young girl brought up with much love, who knew her responsibilities and who could defend herself. They were not worried about me, but they couldn't help checking on me frequently. Living with them, I was a free spirited yet sensible girl. Since I was so severely restrained in my first serious relationship, I was put off men and marriage for a while.

This love affair that turned bad, although very upsetting at that time, would pave the way for a happy marriage later. I regretted having stayed in Turkey to be with him then, but later I would see there is a reason for everything. I felt like a ship seeking a refuge after that stormy relationship, and I would soon find it.

Over two years had passed after that troubling experience. I had pulled myself together. I was working and I travelled often. Free again, I felt so light that I didn't miss having a man in my life, which I filled with work, social activities, and exercise... or maybe the memory of the heavy burden of my last relationship made me avoid a new one. I had been brought up in a modern, open minded family. In Thrace, where women are strong and powerful, I was used to making my own decisions. If I got involved with someone, how could I be happy with a man brought up in a culture of machismo? I didn't feel marriage was for me.

Since I was never going to get married, I was never going to have children. I was probably just as likely to win the lottery as I was to find a suitable spouse. When I felt optimistic, I thought my soul mate was out there somewhere waiting for me. Most of the time, I am a positive thinker, I know how to enjoy little things. I should probably admit that I sometimes beat myself up for little or no reason, as I am given to doing it the hard way. Like my father, I like a challenge, and like my mother, I am a perfectionist; that's what I call double trouble!

It was during that time that I met Ornella, who loved sports like me, and this coincidence was going to change my life. Ornella was a woman pushing 50, but so beautiful and attractive as to make Kim Basinger look dull. We both used to do step aerobics at the Vakkorama gym. At the beginning we only exchanged hellos, then we started to chat a bit, and then we started seeing each other after the gym. I always liked Ornella's view of life. She had a youthful soul and was very lively. Probably because she exercised so much, she was always full of energy, and she was extremely fit. She could have made teenagers jealous with her looks. She was a social butterfly ceaselessly flitting from one place to another; a kind of consular agent for the Italian community in Istanbul, renowned for never missing an activity. It was a pleasure to talk to her on any subject. Furthermore, our chats gave me the opportunity to practice my Italian, which I was afraid of forgetting.

That summer, on August 17, we had the infamous Marmara earthquake, after which we sank into grief as well as a financial crisis. A friend of mine who had a café in Galatasaray was complaining that business was down and asking for my help. As I had quite an entourage in Istanbul, I helped him to organize a few events to bring the place some activity and I asked the renowned painters, cartoonists, and photographers among my friends to paint pictures with coffee as the theme. They indulged me and each gave their interpretations of coffee with beautiful works of art, which we then exhibited on the walls of the café. The exhibition gave new life to the business in the café, and spirits rose.

I have always been a great fan of Italian culture, language, and cuisine. I have seen how every sauce adds a different character to spaghetti, which otherwise seems to be a humble dish. I have enjoyed the local dishes of many different regions and towns and realized there is much more to Italian cuisine than just pizza and pasta. Everybody likes Italian food. Furthermore, there is quite a large Italian client base in Galatasaray as the Italian High school, the Italian Consulate, and the Italian Cultural Association are all located in the area. That's why my friend who knew that coffee is a weak spot for Italians used to serve great Italian coffee in his shop for those who wanted to start the day with an espresso in the morning.

Theme nights are a good formula for cafés and restaurants. We decided to organize an Italian night that would appeal to both Turkish and Italian clients. I don't know where I had found the audacity to cook Italian food for the Italians! I decided to consult Ornella for the menu, who was a skillful cook. When I called her, she said she was having a dinner party that night and invited me to join. I thought to myself, it must be my lucky day! I was going to see how the dishes were prepared, and taste them, too! I took the cook of the café with me and we watched Ornella cook in her kitchen. The party menu was very suitable for our Italian night and we adopted it straight away. I was unaware that the Italian night and my fondness for Italian cuisine would lead me to meet an Italian man, who was going to be the love of my life.

Ornella's dinner guests were arriving. She was greeting them at the door while the cook and I were busy in the kitchen putting the finishing touches on the dishes. When I went into the dining room, an attractive man in an elegant suit came up to me and held out his hand, saying "Ciao!" He seemed to be in his late 30's. I shook his hand and introduced myself. "And I am Cosimo," he said, "we have actually met before." My face felt warm with embarrassment; I am not good at remembering faces and I'm given to committing frequent faux pas. Cosimo turned out to be a friend of Franco's, an Italian friend of mine, whom I had invited to my birthday party four months previous to that in July. He had then asked me if he could bring a friend over, and that friend happened to be Cosimo. What a coincidence it was that we had run across one another again that night at Ornella's. I am both absent-minded and forgetful, and I can imagine myself not paying much attention to someone I had just met when I was celebrating my 29th birthday and had so many of my best friends around. He said he was quite tired that night, too, and had left the party early.

Cosimo worked in an Italian bank in Istanbul, after having worked in Moscow for five years. He had been in Istanbul for two and a half years and seemed to enjoy it. So, through my fondness for Italian food, I ended up meeting the love of my life. They say the way to a man's heart is through his stomach; I find it rather a macho saying, since the same can be said for women. Is it we who choose our destiny or is it our destiny that finds us? I don't know, but after our paths crossed for the second time at Ornella's, Cosimo and I have never been apart since.

Turco-Italian Synthesis[*]

I consider Atilla, a close friend of mine from my university years, who was a civil engineer, to be one of the people who paved the way for our love. He liked to tease me saying architects were of no use and that civil engineers did all the work. I can say I owe it to him to have come across the love of my life. It all started with a dinner party where Atilla almost forced me to go. The two of us were about to go to a movie in Akmerkez when we changed our plans with a phone call I received from Cosimo, whom I had only seen a couple of times until then. He was having a small dinner party at his apartment and he was inviting me to go. When I told him I was in Akmerkez with a friend, he told me to bring him over with me and said he lived just across Akmerkez. Atilla was the one who decided we should go, as I always prefer the movies over anything else. Atilla kept looking for 'the one' to no avail, but he liked to introduce his friends to one another and many couples actually got married thanks to him. He had seen Cosimo once before and thought we suited each other well and believed Cosimo had eyes for me, so he gave me no option but to accept the invitation. He was an engineer and a Chechen man; there was no arguing with him when he got something in his head.

❦

[*] I had connections with interior decoration magazines because of my job. Our apartment with Cosimo was featured in one of the leading magazines, thanks to a friend of mine who worked there. She titled the article "Turco-Italian Synthesis," a phrase which described not only our home, but us as a couple.

Things evolved fast following that dinner party. Cosimo and I had not been together for three months, yet that Sunday morning, while I was still sleepy, he proposed. I must be a very strange woman as I had never dreamed of a man proposing to me on one knee, after a candle-light dinner, with a diamond ring. Therefore, his way of doing it seemed very romantic to me. He was so natural (as he always is), I was splashing cold water on my face at the bathroom sink when he came to me and held me tight, he put a big good morning kiss on my lips and said, "Why don't we get married? We are very happy together. Marry me!" I remember giving a hysterical laugh after a short, stupefied pause. Poor man, what must he have felt! If I had any intention of getting married he definitely would have been the one, but the thought didn't even cross my mind at that time of my life. I think subconsciously I still didn't trust men and was scared. He had been a safe harbor for me after a stormy relationship. I was really happy and peaceful with him, but I guess I needed more time. Also, he was from a different country. I had to go see where he came from and meet his family first. When I told him I didn't want to rush into it, he said, "It's alright, we'll wait as long as you want."

A little while later, his family came to visit him in Istanbul. Among the motives for their visit must have been meeting the girl their son had decided to marry. I will never forget the day I met them; it was a lovely spring morning, we had planned to meet for coffee at the garden of the Four Seasons Hotel. I was very excited to meet the parents of the man I planned to marry. My boyfriend had warned me that his mother was a difficult woman, very critical and hard to please. "She has never approved of any of my girlfriends yet," he said. "I just accept her the way she is. She says what she has to say and I do what I have to do, this is my life and I make my own decisions." I didn't really need to hear this, nervous as I was already. What fault was my boyfriend's exacting mother going to find in me?

I rose early to get prepared, even though it was a Sunday morning. They were waiting for me sitting around a large, round table in the courtyard of the Four Seasons, where inmates must once have paced, as the hotel had been a prison to start with. It was not nearly as bad as I feared. Of course, at the beginning, I felt rather self-conscious as everybody's eyes were on me, but after a while we got used to each other. Cosimo, his mother, his father and his aunt, and I had a nice chat over a cup of cappuccino. Aunty Zia, who had lost her husband at a young age and devoted herself to her sister's children, was present at this significant day as mother number two. I had a typical, sweet Italian family before me! They were warm, friendly people from the south of Italy. They were close-knit family, which was nice, and I could relate to it easily. How similar they were to the Turkish! His mother was an elegant lady of about 60; she was blond with green eyes, and very classy.

We had not known each other for an hour yet when she suddenly turned to me and asked, "So, when are you planning to get married?" I didn't expect the question, Cosimo and I smiled at each other and blurted out, "Very soon." We were both relieved. We had passed the test! His mother had liked me as soon as she had seen me. I could see that Cosimo was surprised as said, "How come everyone, even my mother, likes you?" He later took me to Italy, to the land where he was born and raised. There I fell in love all over again both with him and his country. I had been to Italy many times in the past, I admired it, but I would never have thought I would one day fall in love with an Italian and become an Italian citizen...

Our enjoyable journey to Italy brought us even closer. I came back from it with my mind made up; I was going to build a family with the man I loved. A few months later, in the summer, we held a dinner to celebrate our engagement in the garden of my uncle's farmhouse in Tekirdağ; a long table was dressed, resembling that in the video of Candan Erçetin's song Elbette. I had invited only three friends outside the family; my friend Atilla from the university and Sibel and Ebru, whom I had only known for a year, but was grown very fond of. All three of them came from Istanbul to Tekirdağ to be with me on that day. In fact, the whole thing was Atilla's idea, "I'll take Cosimo to Tekirdağ and we will ask your father for your hand," he said, "it won't do to get married without asking your father. Let the Italian groom see our customs!" I liked the idea, too. The engagement rings were presented on a silver plate, tied to each other with a red ribbon. We put them on and my uncle Kemal cut the ribbon. We had a cozy family ceremony and a nice dinner. A gypsy band called Katil Hasan – Hasan the Murderer – played local tunes and we danced. My cousin Basri was trying to show Cosimo how to belly dance to Thracian music, saying he was "going to naturalize the Italian groom." We were all laughing uncontrollably watching them. I had never dreamed of seeing demure-looking Cosimo dancing to the poignant sound of the Roman clarion. He was having a hard time moving his hands and feet to the rhythm at first, but eventually got the hang of it. Basri and Cosimo's dancing was the highlight of the evening.

We decided to have our wedding in October, which to me is the most beautiful month of autumn. Ornella had to be one of our marriage witnesses, but I couldn't leave my Italian professor Margharita, who had a very special place in my life, out of it, so she had to come from Florence to be one of our witnesses, too. Then there was Libero, Cosimo's childhood friend, and my uncle Mustafa who had hinted that he wished to be one too; so, quite unusually, we had four wedding witnesses instead of two. I don't believe love needs any witnesses at all, but getting married is a formal contract and you have to stick with the formalities even though it may ruin some of the romance.

It Will Get Better Once You Marry

From the very first day of our marriage, Cosimo and I were both enthusiastic about having children. He was the firstborn of an Italian family with three kids and loved children and large families. The sparkle I saw in his eyes whenever there was talk of children made me feel even more eager to have a baby right away. We were both more than ready for it. He was in banking and needed to relocate quite often due to business reasons. He had been in Istanbul for four years now, which meant we would soon have to move out of Turkey. I had a busy work life, too, but I was 30 and Cosimo 38, so we decided to take it up without delay. My periods were irregular and I wanted to know whether it would create a problem. I got an appointment with my regular ob-gyn, Dr. Can, immediately to discuss it.

I had been seeing Dr. Can, who was also my mother's gynecologist, for 16 years. He was a great doctor, who was very kind towards his patients. He was very calm and easy-going. He often called me "my sweet" which instilled peace in me during what can usually be an awkward situation. When I had been to see him for the first time as a teenager he had been very understanding and chatted with me to overcome my nervousness. My experience with him helped me through the bad days I had ahead of me...

During my childhood, Tekirdağ was a small city with a population of less than 50 thousand. Our general practitioner, Dr. Nevres, was of great help to everyone with common complaints such as a cold or flu, but in more serious cases which called for a specialist, the people of Tekirdağ usually didn't trust the specialists in town. Instead, they preferred going to Istanbul for a thorough exam. They used to ask around for a reliable professor and make an appointment with him. Our amiable ob-gyn Dr. Can was always the first choice in gynecological problems for our family and friends living in Tekirdağ. For other troubles we used to ask him to refer us to a good specialist he knew. He was a source of comfort for us.

When I had had my first period at the age of 14, my mother had taken me to see Dr. Can for a checkup and he had been my regular gynecologist ever since. I had stepped into puberty with problems of irregular menstruation, so as I was becoming a woman I was also starting to learn about the problems it brought. Wouldn't it be nice if we could remain children? How troublesome, how painful it is to be a woman! Men are so carefree, they don't have to deal with PMS, menstrual pain, pads, hair removal, dressing up, make-up, and what not. Furthermore, when you are an adolescent you are very irritable and emotional. What you worry about then is not whether your eggs are viable, but your growing breasts and your newly developing curves. It is hard to embrace these changes at the beginning, but in time you start to enjoy them and feel like a woman. When you put on your mother's clothes you don't look like a clown anymore and you've outgrown playing house; you are now a young woman and it's time to rummage through your mother's wardrobe.

During your girlhood you experience identity problems and conflicts with your parents. As your body goes through many changes it can be difficult to adapt to, but eventually you get to accept them all. Some you put up with and some you enjoy. I can say I went through puberty without many problems. I guess I was lucky to have a wholesome circle of friends, among other things. What irritated me most was the increase in hair on my body, especially on my legs, because of which I refused to wear skirts for some time. I don't know if it has anything to do with hair growth, but when we went to see the doctor concerning the irregularity of my periods, he ran some tests and found my prolactin levels too high. I remember using small white pills for about two years to bring them down. Eventually my hormonal level returned to normal, but my legs were still hairy. So I had to accept it as any other change in my body, the silky skin of my childhood was not coming back and I had to visit an aesthetician monthly for a leg wax. My periods were still irregular but my gynecologist told me not to worry about it. "It will all settle down when you get married," he said. But now I was married and my periods had still not settled down. He wasn't right this time!

When my husband and I decided to have a baby in the first

year of our marriage, we discussed this at length with Dr. Can who knew me very well. He said I had an ovulation disorder and I had to take hormone treatments to stimulate my "lazy ovaries." He said, "Why don't we give it a try this month. Start using these hormone pills on the fifth day of your period and we'll see." Were my ovaries to get in shape presently with just one box of pills? Let's assume they did and started to function like clockwork, was I going to get pregnant straightaway? I had so many questions, it was all so unfamiliar to me, but I decided to go along without making a fuss about it. So I did what my doctor recommended and started taking the pills. They gave me hot flashes in the burning hot days of August! Oh my God, this must be how women feel during menopause! Poor mother! I could now understand what she'd been through and why she complained. Later, it turned out that these side effects were due to the dosage that the doctor had prescribed, which was too high for me. I didn't suffer any of it when I took a normal dose.

The summer of 2001 was an unforgettable time for me in many ways. It was the first summer of our marriage. Cosimo wasn't familiar with the Turkish coast yet and I couldn't wait to go swimming with him in my favorite beaches, in the turquoise waters of the Aegean Sea. We spent three weeks travelling the Aegean region and came back with sweet memories. Then I found out I was pregnant. I hadn't expected those tiny hormone pills to work so quickly. I was over the moon.

Losing the Baby

I used to like to let everyone know immediately and celebrate for days whenever I had good news, and that's what I did. They say you shouldn't tell anyone you are pregnant until after the first trimester. But I was so excited that it was impossible for me to keep it a secret. I wanted to scream and let everyone hear it. I invited my best friends over for a party in our apartment; we ate and drank and danced, and celebrated the great news. Cosimo and I were famous for our home parties. We liked to entertain, to give dinner invitations or big parties. Cosimo would play the most popular songs of the day from his collection of over a thousand CDs and at the end of the night we would have had danced so hard that we would be totally exhausted. Since everyone was sure to have fun at our parties; the invitees almost never failed to show up. None of my girlfriends around the same age as me had children yet, so it was all very new to all of us and we didn't know the slightest thing about it. A friend of mine from school brought a children's toy and another friend a pair of baby socks to the party. My husband said that in Italy they believed it brought bad luck to get things for a baby before it was born. Now, Italians are even more superstitious than we Turks! I couldn't believe Cosimo could fret about something like that, open minded as he normally was, but he had beliefs coming from his childhood.

When the baby was only five weeks old, I went to see Dr. Can for my first prenatal exam. He did an ultrasound, but it was too early, yet, and there wasn't much to be seen. Normally one should wait until after the seventh week for the first visit, but I was so excited that I kept showering Dr. Can with questions.

He answered each of them patiently and thoroughly, but he also warned me against getting too excited and said we would learn more about the baby in a few weeks' time. Meanwhile, with the influence of the people around me, I decided to change my doctor and got an appointment with Dr. Alp, an ob-gyn specialist. He was well known as the IVF specialist for Turkish actress and pop star Hülya Avşar's. At that time he was only renowned for his successful professional career and he wasn't yet being stalked by the paparazzi as he later would be. Waiting for my appointment I was eyeing the reception area of his practice, as luxuriously decorated as the lobby of the Çırağan Hotel, and thinking, 'So this is how it is to be the ob-gyn of celebrities. He must have something over the doctors I've seen so far if he is this well-off!'

Finally, I was in. The doctor was doing the ultrasound and I was holding my breath watching the baby, or a blurred figure, more precisely, on a giant screen hanging from the ceiling. I could hear the heartbeat on a device with speakers like a stereo; it reminded me of a galloping horse, thubalup, thubalup... My poor heart was bursting with emotion, it was an unutterable happiness; I had a living being inside me, God, how lucky I was! I remember having a moment's distress: I was facing a responsibility of a lifetime. Was I going to be a good mother? But it was too early to think about all this. I was over the moon. It was a shame Cosimo was not there to share this moment with me, how excited he would have been if he could have been there. I had to bring him to the next appointment.

While I was getting dressed, the doctor had taken his seat on a high-backed chair behind the stylish desk. When I went and sat on the patient's seat, he first asked me questions about my medical history. I told him all the problems I had in my teenage years in great detail while he listened without making any comments or asking questions. Then he answered my countless questions concisely, almost curtly, which I didn't care for. Maybe this was normal, I was after all a new patient, and perhaps it took time for doctors to feel comfortable with a patient, too. The only other gynecologist I had known before was Dr. Can, who could count as a family friend, so it was not surprising that we should have a cordial dialogue.

I was so happy that nothing could put me off. I had a single thought in mind: my baby. I kept dreaming of holding it in my arms. When I went back to the doctor's again in two weeks, I had my friend Erika with me, who had come from Florence to see us. Cosimo had to miss it again as the appointment time was during business hours. I didn't mind, thinking we still had seven months to go, he would come to one of the many subsequent appointments we had ahead of us. Erika was a close friend, almost like a family member. I insisted that she go in with me, I wanted her to hear the baby's heartbeat. Happiness doubles when shared, I wanted to share my happiness with her as Dr. Alp didn't seem too keen on sharing.

My classy doctor was working on the sonogram, trying to work out how far along I was. "It's your ninth week," he said. How time stalled! This was my third appointment in the course of four weeks, I was so excited and impatient. Erika and I were staring at the screen, waiting for what the doctor had to say. "There is no heartbeat," Dr. Alp said, without so much as the shadow of any emotion in his face. I couldn't believe it; I didn't want to believe it. I must be a bad dream! My eyes met Erika's. We were stunned.

The doctor went on: "The embryo is no longer alive, this is a miscarriage. You need to have an abortion. Come to the American Hospital tomorrow morning. You will be anaesthetized, so don't eat or drink anything. You won't need to stay in the hospital overnight; you will be discharged the same day..."

But I could hardly listen; I was stuck at the very first sentence, still unable to grasp it fully. It was like a bad dream, but, alas, I was awake! "How can this be, doctor?" I stuttered. "Did I do something wrong? Is it something I did?"

"No, it's just natural selection," he answered. The unhealthy, weak embryo aborts itself. It won't make it. I'm sorry for your loss."

You never expect bad things to happen to you. And there are some things in life you just don't expect might ever come your way, a miscarriage was one of those things for me. My dreams of motherhood came crumbling down. I asked myself, for the first time at the age of 31, the question I was to ask many times in the six years to come: 'Was I ever going to be able to be a mother?'

When, still drowsy from anesthesia, I opened my eyes after the operation, I saw two bald men on my left and right staring at me. I remember thinking I had double vision for a moment. After a few seconds, when I could see better, I realized the handsome man on my right was my husband and the other one was my doctor. After Dr. Alp asked me how I felt and left, my husband leaned over me and planted a kiss on my lips. Caressing my hand, "Don't worry," he said, trying to comfort me, "everything is going to be alright. You are the only one that matters at this moment, you and your health."

You know how you try to find someone to blame when you are overwhelmed by grief. When I lost the baby – even though I knew it was absurd – I thought it was because of 'evil eyes' as I had been so enthusiastic to spread the news. When you are sick with sadness, you think of all kinds of weird, stupid things. Cosimo blamed it on the early baby gifts. To comfort him and myself, the first thing I did was to buy an amulet to fend off bad eyes and to give away the presents. I remember feeling empty for some time after the miscarriage. It was as if I was an empty shell, something had fallen away from inside me, a fetus had come to life in my womb for a very short time, only to die and leave me unexpectedly. It was as if I had lost a bit off my heart. I had a lump in my throat that I could only dissolve by crying, and when I wasn't able to cry it got bigger and harder and choked me.

Postabortion Blues

I was weary, helpless, empty and beaten. For a long time, I didn't want to do anything. I forced myself to go into bookstores to browse the shelves, to go to movies to see romantic comedies, or to sit in a café to leaf through a magazine; to try and lift my mood. These activities were lifesavers that I clung to when I felt low. During my high school or university years, when I was under stress because of projects or exams, I used to yield to eating mindlessly and put on weight, which was bad for me. Fortunately, I had given this bad habit up after I started to work and I had learned to find other healthier ways to feel better. I've always found browsing the shelves of bookstores is a kind of meditation to me and felt that I can let go of my thoughts when I am engrossed in a book. I wanted to read about pregnancy losses, but I couldn't find any books in Turkish about this topic, although there were quite a number in other languages. Had no one in Turkey ever wanted to write about such an important a subject for a woman? A miscarriage was a failure, a defeat, a breakdown. Yes, it might be a private thing for a woman, perhaps many women liked to keep it to themselves, but women had to know they were not alone when they went through this. Sharing might alleviate their heartache. That was my doctor's advice to me: Talk about it, get it off your chest.

At that time I didn't have any friends who had had a similar experience nor anyone to talk about it. I had to go through it alone. I thought it would go away with time; I tried to forget it and not to make a big deal out of it. But the same pain I had buried inside me would come back all over again in two years.

I had left that misfortune behind and assumed my usual busy pace; I was focusing on my job. After a while I felt I was physically and emotionally well again. I felt strong enough to go back to pursuing my dream of having a baby. I talked to Cosimo, my darling husband and best friend, and we decided to try again. Just then we heard from the headquarters of the Italian bank where Cosimo worked that they planned on assigning him to a position in Shanghai. China was far away but it could be interesting to live there. There was a period of uncertainty. We decided it would be best to hold off our plan of having a baby for a while so it wouldn't coincide with moving. The appointment became final towards the end of 2002; we were to move to Barcelona in Spain instead of China. We were both very happy about it. Spain was a lovely country and it was close to both Turkey and Italy. I was so busy with organizing the move that it didn't even occur to me to feel sad about leaving my country. It was all like a game, a new country, a new home, a new life, it was so exciting. In March 2003, as the ship carrying all our things left Istanbul for Barcelona, we packed a few suitcases in our car and started our 15-day, 3,000-kilometer journey for the same destination.

2

Barcelona

I opened my eyes in an unpleasant, grim hospital room. For a
moment I couldn't recall why I was there. What had happened to
me? I tried to pull it together; my mind was numb with anesthesia.
When his warm hand grasped mine I felt an instant relief. It didn't
matter where I was, my darling was there, and I was safe...

"Good morning," he said with his affectionate voice. "Are you
alright, amore?" I wasn't so sure I was alright, I was numb all over.
I couldn't move my hands, but I said I was alright to comfort him.
He had obviously been worrying about me all night, you could see
from his bloodshot eyes that he hadn't slept. Last night's incidents
were now coming back to me. We had both had a terrible fright.

Did I have to suffer that much? My emotional loss was more
than I could take. I had had another miscarriage. This had been
worse as I had a spontaneous abortion. This was the second defeat
on my way to having a baby. That night, I wasn't only emotionally,
but also physically broken. I still shivered when I remembered the
pain and terror I'd experienced for about an hour until I could
make it to the hospital from home and be given an injection for

the pain.

A cross hung on the wall over the bed. This answered my questions. I was in a Catholic hospital. Catholic faith opposes abortion. My pregnancy was terminated, but according to the hormone levels in the blood I was still considered pregnant. The doctor in charge hadn't even bothered giving me a sonogram. A baby couldn't be removed from the mother's womb in a Catholic hospital even when its heart had stopped beating, the mother's body had to expel it by itself. So I was left to have a miscarriage...

I was surprised that such a method could still be used today, it seemed extremely primitive to me to let a dead baby lie in a woman's womb, to wait for her body to expel it by itself. I felt it was cruel, the worst thing you could do to a woman who had just lost her baby. It was torture, both emotionally and physically. I didn't know the city yet, I was in a place of which I wasn't familiar with either the language or the culture. I hadn't so much as imagined such things could happen to me in a hospital that I had chosen because of its proximity to where we lived and thinking it was a good one. There was nothing to do, I had my hands tied.

That day, I hated being a foreigner in Barcelona...

The Surprise Party

Warm and friendly, Jill was a naturalized Turk who spoke Turkish fluently and she was a close friend of mine. I felt I had known her for years even though we'd only met two and a half years ago. She was American; she'd fallen in love with a Turkish architect and moved to Istanbul to get married to him. Her father was a German man who had moved to the US years before. Jill had nothing to do with the 'foreign brides' in Turkey who complained continuously. She loved Turkey and Turkish people. She had combined her German-American genes nicely with the Turkish spirit.

We had met in a hotel in Uludağ, waiting in line for the open buffet with our plates at hand. We had a lot in common and both of us were in love with skiing. Jill had been skiing almost since she was born. Whereas, I had learned to at the age of 21, she had been part of the junior Olympic ski team in the US until she had a knee injury. I had never skied anywhere but in the short ski tracks in Turkey; she raced down in a flash with agile movements while I tried to work out the safest way down. Nevertheless, we were equally fond of skiing and we had great fun in spite of the difference between our skill levels. Jill, her husband Kerem, and Cosimo and I made a great quartet. Heavy snow had buried our bus (and all other vehicles), forcing us to extend our holiday. We spent the time where we waited for it to clear to ski some more and to get to know each other further. Two days flew by unnoticed with cheerful conversation and we grew closer to one another. When the bus was still stuck after two days we decided to find some other way to go back to Istanbul, which we did via a journey full of adventure. The ski holiday was over, but our friendship wasn't and we kept in touch in Istanbul.

When we were to relocate to Barcelona, Jill was among those who got most upset about it. She was one of my friends I saw most often, we had a beautiful friendship. We were going to miss each other.

I had so many friends I wanted to say goodbye to before moving to Barcelona! I didn't know if I was going to manage to see everyone and I had mentioned it to Jill once. She was a very thoughtful person and had immediately started to think about something to make my wish come true. Her husband Kerem was an interior architect and had recently decorated a restaurant in Beyoğlu, called Şarabi, which was famous for its wine selection. We had been meaning to taste their wines and see our friend Kerem's work. Jill had made a reservation with the restaurant and organized a surprise party with the help of Sibel, a close friend of mine, who had the numbers of all my friends, old and new. My husband, Jill, and Sibel had managed to keep it from me until the last day, when Nesli let it slip. I had met Nesli in Aşk Café to say goodbye; I thought it was going to be our last meeting for some time as we were to leave for Barcelona in a few days. So, I held her tight when saying farewell and said, "God knows when I'll see you again."

To which she just replied, "I'll see you tomorrow night at your party at Şarabi." I had – unfortunately – found out about the surprise party, but I didn't let anyone know.

That night, we met with Ornella at the bar of the Pera Palas Hotel – which hadn't been restored yet and was almost falling apart, but I liked the bar and the pastry shop – to have drink before dinner. After we drank a couple rather strong cocktails, Ornella came up with an idea and she told us she knew a nice restaurant in Beyoğlu, where we could have dinner and carry on with our conversation, to which we all agreed. So, this had to be the venue for the surprise party.

When, going down the stairs inside the restaurant to the dim tavern at the basement floor, I found my beloved friends waiting for me and I burst into tears. Frankly, I hadn't thought a surprise, which I had found out before time, would move me that much. It was a great moment to see everyone I loved together and I can never forget it in my life. It was a lovely night with more of my friends there than I could count, we ate and drank and danced, we laughed and cried, it was both merry and sentimental. Jill had done a great job. At the end of the night, I put my purse filled with notes, cards, letters, and gifts from my friends into my suitcase without looking inside.

I read everything they'd written the next day in the car while we were waving goodbye to Turkey and entering Greece via Ipsala border checkpoint, with tears rolling down my cheeks. We have since moved five more times and each time we threw away lots of stuff, but I've never even dreamed of parting with these letters, which I still keep dearly.*

Farewell To My Homeland From Ipsala

Even though at first it seemed like a game to leave my parents, my brother, my friends and relatives, my baby that I'd lost, my country, my home, my childhood, my youth, my schools, my job, Istanbul, Tekirdağ, the Marmara Sea – basically everything that had shaped me – behind and to sail away towards a new life, as the road drove me away from my loved ones and the number of miles in between

---

* We thought of Jill and Kerem as a sweet couple and suddenly we heard that they'd split up. Jill moved back to the US (even though she loved Turkey) because she wasn't able to find a suitable job. Kerem remained in Istanbul. As they don't have children, they've never seen each other since.

kept increasing I felt as though I was losing something inside and couldn't keep tears from swelling in my eyes. I didn't wish to upset my husband, who already felt guilty for tearing me apart from my country, so I fought back the tears. I am very sentimental and cry easily, and today I had more than enough reason to cry. I was leaving my country and going overseas.

The reason we had decided to go to Barcelona by car was our wish to turn it into a journey. The plan was to drive to Barcelona from Istanbul through Greece, Italy, and France, in a trip that should take roughly 15 days. After setting off from Istanbul, we first stopped in Tekirdağ to see my parents. From there we drove to the Greek border under heavy March snow falling over Thrace. We went through Greece to the Gulf of Patras. From the Port of Patras we took the ferry to the Puglia region of Italy, where my husband had been born. So, Puglia was to Cosimo what Thrace was to me, his family, his roots were there. He had been living away from his family for over 20 years, but he had never forgotten where he was from and never forgotten his family. We went to see his family and did some catching up.

We couldn't miss a visit to Florence to see some old friends and enjoy the amazing Tuscan cuisine. That gorgeous Renaissance city captures me with a different detail every time I visit it. We left unwillingly to go to San Remo, on the Ligurian coast known as 'Italy's Côte d'Azur,' one of those places offering not only historical treasures but also great natural beauty. San Remo is known for its annual music festival. My dear friend Rebi had offered us the weekend package he had won as a gift from a hotel in San Remo, so we decided to visit this musical province on our way. We had a lovely weekend in San Remo, after which we left Italy's Ligurian coast for France's famous Côte d'Azur.

Although it was March, the weather was nice and warm at the Mediterranean coast of France. France was breathtakingly beautiful. We saw Nice and Cannes. We visited Monaco, the rich but tiny country. Then we went through provinces such as Avignon and Arles which have inspired world-famous artists like van Gogh and Picasso with their beauty and Montpellier which was a lovely province close to the Spanish border, to finally arrive at Barcelona, which we entered through the impressive 'Avenue Diagonale,' with giant palm trees on the median strip and elegant shops on both sides, that cuts diagonally through the city. When made it to our hotel that night, we were already in love with Barcelona.

Barcelona, Barcelona

Barcelona, which has quite a history, is said to have lived its first golden era between the 13th and 15th centuries and its second one during the 1992 Olympic Games. I wouldn't know about the first episode, but I sure remember the second one, having witnessed how it helped Barcelona flourish. Before then, Spain had taken one of the best decisions in its history by joining the European Union, before which it was a poor country with a rich cultural heritage. I remember that in 1988, when we went for a tour of Europe with my friends, it required no visa to enter Spain while all the other European countries required one. Yet, we didn't include Spain in our tour because we had limited time and Spain lay quite outside our route as well as because Spain was then known as a "not-so-civilized" country. It turns out I had in my fate not only to visit, but to live in this country.

The 1992 Olympic Games touched Barcelona like a magic wand. The city became a shining star and grew into the fashion, entertainment, style, and design center of Western Europe almost overnight. Its unique blend of Mediterranean and Catalan cultures fuelled its unstoppable rise. The city was dressed up; the municipality emphasized urban design and invested generously in the beaches. Clean, sandy beaches right at the center of the city where entertainment lasted through the night was so appealing to the youth that Amsterdam lost favor and students or post-school tourists started to favor Barcelona. It became every university student's dream to go to Barcelona via the Erasmus student exchange program.

Barcelona made it to the list of the cities with the highest living standards and eventually became the favorite holiday spot of rich tourists as well as the young travelers. Today, the posh stores of famous brands are chock-full of Japanese, American, and Russian tourists. Many people who come for a business trip fall in love with the city and settle there. Foreigners with artistic tendencies who come with cultural tours or attend art schools here adore Barcelona. There are gourmets who come exclusively for gastronomic trips; the restaurants swarm with clients thanks to their world-famous chefs. Ferran Adria, who was selected the best chef of the world a few years ago with his discovery of molecular cuisine is from a town close to Barcelona. You used to have to book a year earlier if you wanted to eat in his restaurant in the city, El Bulli, and you would have to pay a bill of roughly 250 Euros per person. Ferran Adria must have had his fill of money and fame apparently, as he closed the place down, but the chefs who worked under him each have their own places now, thriving on his legacy.

I've heard that Ferran Adria, apparently fed up with the restaurant business, has ventured into brewing and is working on creating an exclusive beer brand to compete with the British.

Barcelona is a real design paradise! All the buildings' façades are the work of famous architects. In the streets the benches, lamp posts, the paving stones, the balustrades, the fountains, the toilets, everything you can think of are the work of famous designers. Magnificent historical mansions adorn the vast, stylish avenues. The patrons of the street cafés sit under the cool shade of linden trees. The windows of the elegant stores compete with one another in style. All the brands of the world are here, none are missing! The days are rather hot in summer, but in the other seasons the mild Mediterranean climate prevails, making life easy and the city delightful. In Barcelona, people live their life almost entirely out on the streets. There are people who don't ever use the kitchen in their homes. I remember having a hard time while we were looking for an apartment to rent. The Spanish don't make a fuss about the interior of their homes, probably because they like living outside. The city is designed to suit pedestrians, it's a pleasure to walk here, unlike in Turkey where the sidewalks are either non-existent or two feet high, turning a walk in the street into an ordeal! Here even the traffic lights are pedestrian friendly, you don't have to hurry when you are crossing the street, and the green light stays on for a long time so people can cross leisurely. Cars wait patiently and traffic jams are rare. It's almost too good to be true and fun to watch.

Barcelona is an exemplary city from the city planning perspective and is taught as a case study in architectural schools in universities. In 1998, when a new project was to be done for

Istanbul Atatürk Airport, the famous architectural firm GMW from Britain had opened an office in Istanbul, moving almost the entire firm there. I had met Mr. Ali Özveren, the architect in charge of the project, then, and he'd become a friend, whose opinion I valued dearly. When I told him that I was to move to Barcelona, "Lucky you," he said. "You are going to a paradise for architects. It's a beautiful city where you will come across very few eyesores. It's a city that stays awake almost 24 hours, although to a lesser extent than Istanbul, but it's so much less chaotic and the living standards are much higher." Then he went on to say, "When I visited there, what I liked most was that in the buildings in the city center life never stops, it goes on day and night. The ground floors are usually occupied by tapas bars, cafés, restaurants or stores. The first floors house offices and the higher floors are residential. So the building is always awake and bustling, the energy never dwindles."

I was to experience firsthand how right he was.

Like all good things in life, Barcelona has its own little flaw: There are two languages spoken here. Everything, even street names, are written in two languages. Now, maybe this is a trait rather than a flaw. I have nothing against there being two languages, but I cannot quite understand how Catalan prevails over Spanish even though we arc in Spain. When you go to a public office, a community clinic or a hospital, the forms you are handed to fill are in Catalan, which is not fair; if, as a foreign resident, you have managed to learn Spanish should you still have to learn Catalan? And I'm not the only one who complains; even the Spanish citizens coming from other parts of the country find it difficult.

You begin to understand how strong this 'Catalan-ism' is only when you start to mingle with the city's daily life... Judging from the graffiti on the walls of the buildings and bus stops, the people here wish for Catalan to be the sole language in this region. They even seem to think people other than Catalans should not be here at all. My husband and I used to go to the cinema quite often to see foreign movies in their original language. We witnessed Catalans protesting even this, crying "We want movies in Catalan!" It's not only the language, the Catalans exaggerate it a bit and want to declare their independence. Now, that is Barcelona's flaw. Even if you live here for years you always feel you're an alien because you cannot speak Catalan and the Catalans always exclude you. Except for that Catalan-ism, I think Barcelona is one of the best cities on earth to live in. If, like many other foreigners who fell in love with and moved to Barcelona, you don't make a fuss about it and choose to enjoy what the city has to offer, then it is the perfect city with its sandy beaches, its sea, its mountains, forests, history and architecture.

It's the Right City To Have a Baby!

A few months after we settled in our new home in Barcelona and got used to the city, we were convinced it was the ideal place to have a baby. Not that it really mattered to us; even if we had settled in a bachelors' city like New York or Paris, it probably wouldn't have stopped us from going ahead with our plans of having children, but Barcelona was really inspiring and we felt like making babies.

Barcelona is a real family city with its nice and moderate

climate, clean, sandy beaches right in the city, and its lovely trees and parks... Wherever you look in the streets, you see parents or grandparents or nannies pushing strollers, each family has two or three, or even four kids. The Spanish outdo Italians in family size. Italian families have been growing smaller in recent years due to the country's economic struggles and high cost of living, and many families have a single child. Yet another important characteristic of Barcelona is its exemplary urban design. Everything has been meticulously planned for comfortable living: train and subway stations have elevators or ramps; there are cycle lanes and tracks, play grounds for children of various age groups at each corner (it's unbelievable, play grounds are divided into three separate areas for different age groups); restaurants and cafés offer special children's menus, high-chairs, play areas, nursing and changing rooms... Everything is there to serve the needs of families with children.

After painfully unpacking the last of our nearly two hundred boxes in the summer heat we decided we had earned a holiday. We were with my family in Turkey. The sea was beautiful and it felt so good to swim. We thought we were ready to act again to make our dream of having a baby (postponed because of the hustle and bustle of moving) come true. When I went to Istanbul, I went to see Dr. Can and told him I wanted to try again. Once more, he prescribed the selfsame little white hormone pills as in my earlier pregnancy, to stimulate the lazy ovaries. He wished me luck and I came back to our new home in Barcelona with the pills in my suitcase.

I waited impatiently for my period. In the meantime, I had to visit the community health center in our neighborhood to have an injection that Dr. Can had prescribed back in Turkey for a yeast infection he had diagnosed, to be on the safe side before pregnancy. I was now a resident of Barcelona and could benefit from the health services... If I could manage to fill out a form, which was, of course, in Catalan. The form in Spanish had to be especially requested. As for the injection, in Spain, you cannot have a pharmacist or a medic to inject you with just any shot you request. Since the nurses asked for the translation of Dr. Can's prescription into Spanish, I couldn't get my shot nor fill out the form and have a health services card issued.

The summer of 2003 was disastrously hot. I could never forget the heat rising from the molten asphalt brushing my face like the flames of a fire every time I stepped out of the building. The real estate agent who had rented us the apartment had warned us that it had no air conditioning, but my husband and I didn't mind, and had ignored his advice. What a mistake! That summer, in that hellish heat, we regretted renting an apartment without AC as it was impossible to breathe inside, let alone sleep! It was an exceptionally hot summer with temperatures much higher than the seasonal averages. In Barcelona the weather is usually hot like in Izmir, but that summer was extraordinary, it was not hot, but searing hot. It was no use leaving the windows open at night, there was not the slightest breeze. Not that it was possible to sleep through the noise of the Spanish people who sleep during the day and play during the night anyway! Add to that the hormone pills I was taking, it was as if I had a volcanic eruption in my body. The hot flashes middle age women have during menopause must be something like that. I was on fire. When I took my temperature, it was normal, but I felt like a 100 degrees Celsius.

Dr. Can must have decided to give my ovaries a real boost and given me too high a dose, because when I had used the same pills for the first time two years ago, although it was also in August, I hadn't experienced anything like this. With the heat wave on top of my hot flashes, we had to get away somewhere cooler. A short holiday together would also give us more time to make babies. We found out that the only rainy region then was the Basque region in the north of Spain. We packed quickly and left the next day. The Basque region was already on our list of places to see anyway, I had been wishing to see the Guggenheim Museum in Bilbao since I had studied architecture and Cosimo was as enthusiastic about modern architecture.

I had found us a nice little romantic boutique hotel at the foot of the mountain in San Sebastian where we stayed, it was a well-kept villa surrounded by lush gardens, run as hotel by a family. Spain is unmatched in tourism; they are so good at it. Small hotels are very stylish, clean and comfortable. You eat very well even in the most unpretentious restaurant. Spain is a great country with its history, its culture, its cuisine, its climate, its sea and sun! In the meantime, I had gone through my little white pills and was nearing my productive days. Perfect timing, perfect ambiance, things couldn't get better. Even the weather was on our side, I can't recall any other occasions I've enjoyed rain so much. Rain was refreshing us up after the searing heat of Barcelona. We toured San Sebastian, a city renowned for its beaches and tapas bars. We went for a gastronomic tour in the city of Bilbao famous for its chefs. And we visited Frank O. Gery's magnificent Guggenheim Museum, which left us in awe. We took our hat off to the Spanish once again. It was not in vain that their country was flooded with tourists every year, they knew how to turn even the most ordinary of cities into a focal point for tourists by supporting big projects that add value to a city. Cities where no one would set foot gained popularity with modern architectural buildings. When I see such places, I can't help fretting about the fact that you never see a famous architect realizing a project in Istanbul, Ankara or İzmir. What does Bilbao have that, say, Trabzon, which is also in the north, rainy and green, doesn't? This brings out the nationalist in me and these questions keep turning in my head...

Here I Am, Pregnant Again!

My period is late! My periods are not all that regular, so at first I don't really notice but then I start wondering if I am pregnant... I have no patience to wait; I get a pregnancy test from a pharmacy at once. When I was pregnant for the first time in Turkey, I went to the doctor straight away and had a blood test, so it's my first time with those home-pregnancy-tests. I look at the large box in my hand; turn it over a few times. Is it because of my poor Spanish or is it really complicated? I don't know, but I can't figure out how to use the stick with little pink and blue windows on it. With a little help from the dictionary and with persistent determination, I finally grasp it; it's actually quite simple, all you need to do is to put a few drops of your urine on the stick.

Whoever it is who writes the pamphlets for the pharmaceutical companies, they are definitely brilliant at making it look complicated! I take the test and wait. It says in the leaflet that it might take a few minutes for the lines on the stick to appear. One minute or two can seem so long! But, what is it?! Suddenly two lines appear. I can't believe I got it right. Two lines showing, does it really mean that I am pregnant? According to the figure on the paper, yes, it does. But I'd better have Cosimo read it; too, Italians are better at understanding Spanish. Cosimo confirms it. I got it alright. My darling husband and I embrace and whisper tender words to each other, we pray for everything to go smoothly this time. It's too early to see a doctor yet, but I call Dr. Can in Istanbul and let him know of the situation. He says he is happy for me and asks me to keep him informed.

Cosimo is hopeful, while I am anxious. I know that having had a miscarriage the first time doesn't mean I'll lose the baby this time as well, but I can't help worrying about it.

❦

We had chosen an apartment in the city center in Barcelona, on a lovely square with many cafés and restaurants. I've always found the squares in Mediterranean cities very attractive. When I was in Italy to learn the language, I used to like to study in the cafés in several 'piazzas.' I like the idea of being able to socialize as soon as you set your foot out of your door and I had always dreamed of living in a home on a square like that. We contacted a real estate agent and looked at several apartments that met our criteria. We saw that in Spain, the same apartment could be shown by more than one agent, which we found a little odd. We decided to go on our search for an apartment independently from one another to speed up the process. Cosimo looked at apartments during his lunch break every day, and I, all day – except, of course, the four-hour siesta from 1 to 5 o'clock – and we evaluated the findings of the day in the evening, sharing the pros and cons of the apartments we'd seen. We saw a total of 45 apartments between the two of us.

It was not an easy job to find a new or well-kept apartment to rent in Barcelona. One evening, talking about the apartments we'd seen that day, we realized we had both seen and liked the same one. Obviously, since we were both impressed by the same apartment among so many, it was the right one for us. It was in a building with a historical façade and a renovated, modern interior, it was very comfortable and stylish, and I'd fallen in love with it at first sight.

There was a hospital just across our building on Plaza Molina that we'd heard was a good one. I thought it was a good idea to go to a hospital nearby, at least for the first months of my pregnancy, I trusted Spanish healthcare. What was the worst thing that could happen? If I wasn't satisfied, I could always change hospitals. So I registered with the hospital and I was assigned to an ob-gyn who happened to be available at that moment. I first had a blood test, which confirmed my pregnancy. During the first appointment, I gave the doctor my detailed medical history, including the drugs and therapies I had taken, my hormonal condition and my periods. I was afraid of having another miscarriage, so I asked him – or maybe begged him– to take any precautionary measures possible before it was too late. From a medical perspective, I wasn't yet considered a risky case as I had had only one miscarriage. You shouldn't be pessimistic, but why should you wait for something bad to happen if you can take precautions beforehand?

After our interview (half English, half Spanish and even partly Catalan), the doctor performed an ultrasound scan. I was only five weeks pregnant and it was too early to say anything. You couldn't even hear the heartbeat before the seventh or eighth week. But everything seemed normal so far. My husband and I shared a kiss of joy after the visit. I wasn't too sure I liked the doctor, but then, it was only the first visit. It was not easy to communicate with a doctor whose language I didn't speak and who didn't speak English very well. He hadn't given heed to what I said, but I didn't know whether it was because he couldn't understand very well or because he didn't really care. Women like a doctor who talks to us, comforts us and tells us everything in detail. It's not easy to find a doctor with whom you can communicate, especially when, like me, you have just moved to a new country where you don't know anybody, don't speak the language, and have to select a doctor randomly.

This time, I wasn't going to tell anyone I was pregnant, not even my mother. I had been very precocious in my first pregnancy and told everybody, this time I was going to be prudent, but it was really hard for me. Often I had to bite my lips not to tell. A very close friend of mine from the university, Elif, was to come to Spain on an architectural tour of Valencia and Barcelona. I invited her over to dinner one night when she was there. I kept myself from sharing the news even with her, although I wanted to so badly. We decided to meet the next day to visit some of the works of Gaudi, the famous architect, which was already on the program of the group she was with. I wanted to show her the communication tower built by Frank O. Ghery on a hill with a bird's eye view on the city. Although not many tourists visited the tower, part of it was open to visitors, with an entrance fee. Now, Barcelona municipality was very good at marketing the city and their most important income source was tourism. While we were exploring the tower, it suddenly occurred to me that we were on a transmitting station with antennae all around and that the radio waves could hurt the baby. I shuddered with alarm and told Elif I had to go out immediately. I made off and found myself downstairs. My friend Elif thoughtfully refrained from asking any questions and soon joined me downstairs. I don't know if she would still remember that day, but I can never forget it, the few minutes on the tower felt like horror movie come to life. I was nursing my precious load; I was ready to do anything to keep it out of harm's way.

Yet Another Miscarriage

I had a strange feeling. I keep telling myself it's just anxiety; there is nothing to worry about. But I had a feeling that it's not going to work, that I'm going to lose this baby, too.

I didn't feel pregnant at all. My breasts, which had grown fuller and harder were back to their normal size, the swelling of my body was reduced. There was something wrong, I could feel it. I couldn't wait until the next visit, set to take place on the seventh week, with this nagging doubt. I called the doctor and asked for an appointment, but he told me that it would be unnecessary and that I should have a blood test done. I had the test, which indicated that I was still pregnant. But I knew from books that pregnancy hormones might still be present in the body even though the embryo might have died. But why didn't the doctor bother to give me at least an ultrasound scan? I was really nervous. I went to the hospital a few times, talked to the doctor's assistant and insisted on having an appointment, banging doors when I had to leave empty handed. I was powerless, helpless, and desperate. I knew I was losing the baby (if I hadn't already lost it), but there was nothing I could do about it, the doctor just wouldn't lift a finger!

✤

We'd found out by coincidence that a friend of Cosimo's from the years when he worked in Moscow also lived in Barcelona with his family and we had met for dinner a couple of times. Aldo and his kind family did everything they could so we wouldn't feel on our own in Barcelona. They had introduced us to their circle of friends. Aldo's wife Laura had introduced me to Angelica, who was a saint. She is a strong, kind, friendly woman and mother of three. I was having one of my bad days when she called and invited me to go to the swimming pool of the gym to which she belonged. It also had a bath, a sauna, a spa and a beauty center. This normally should have been an irresistible invitation for me as I am a Cancer and I love playing with water, but I didn't feel comfortable with the idea of going into a pool as I had doubts about my pregnancy. When Angelica insisted, I decided to share my concerns with her. I hadn't told anyone of my pregnancy yet, but I really needed to share it with someone as it was preying on my mind. In the meantime, I had started to have a pink discharge, which wasn't a good sign. Not that I'd experienced anything like this before; the first time I'd had a miscarriage the doctor had seen it on the ultrasound and arranged for me to have an operation the next day.

It was obvious I wasn't going anywhere with this doctor; so I got an appointment from the Dexeus University Hospital renowned for their scientific research studies. We went with Cosimo, in the evening after he finished work. I could see a black dot in the ultrasound, but no movement. The doctor – thank God he spoke English – told us there was no heartbeat and that an abortion was required. It was Monday, the operation was scheduled for Wednesday morning and I was told to report to the hospital without eating anything in the morning. I was very sad but it was nothing like the shock I'd had the first time, I was better prepared for the bad news, I'd probably known it for days. My dear husband Cosimo was trying to comfort me. When we got back home, he sat me on the couch and asked me what I'd like to have for dinner. I felt like some spaghetti pomodoro. Cosimo put some music on and lit the candles to cheer me up and disappeared in the kitchen, from where mouthwatering aromas were soon to emanate.

Half way through the meal, I felt a shooting pain in my pelvis. I sprang up from my chair and scurried to the bathroom. Labor pain must be something like that. I was doubled over with pain. Then I felt a warm gush of blood down my legs. I was having a spontaneous abortion, just like I dreaded. It was because of the strict Catholic rules that I was having to go through this. With great difficulty, I walked to the hospital across the square in my pajamas, with Cosimo's help, as the university hospital was a 20 minutes' drive, which there was no way I could make.

Drenched in blood, I was admitted to the ER. Almost an hour elapsed before I was given a shot of pain killers, every minute of which was torture. "Deliver me," I cried in revolt against those who put me through this. "Deliver me at once, save me from this agony!" But they said I couldn't be anaesthetized as I had just eaten and I had to wait for next morning. Another reason they couldn't proceed immediately was that the abortion could only be performed by my own doctor! I couldn't believe I would have to put up with this when I didn't even want to see his face anymore! It was too late to do anything else, so we waited for the morning in that grim hospital room with my husband.

The next morning, when I opened my eyes, I was in this same room. I touched my belly, trying to recall the events of the past night. I had lost my baby... again.

Second Defeat

It takes only a few days for a woman's body to recover after a miscarriage. Physically, I felt alright, but emotionally, I didn't think I could recover that easily. I felt like a defeated warrior. The doctors said that the uterus would be ready for a new pregnancy after the next period following the miscarriage. I found it amazing that the body could bounce back in such a short time period and wondered at its resilience, but the body's healing is one thing, the mind's is another.

I decided to give myself some time before trying again. I was scared; I didn't want to go through the same thing all over again if I got pregnant once more. I couldn't help asking "Why me?" I knew that one in every ten pregnancies end up with a miscarriage, in other words there was a ten percent risk of loss in every pregnancy, but did I have to be in that ten percent every time?

Miscarriage is a very common condition, and quite devastating for a woman. Most miscarriages take place before the 12th week of the pregnancy and most women can hardly enjoy the first trimester because they feel threatened by the risk of loss. This is why pregnant women usually keep it to themselves for the first three months!

I kept reading everything I could get my hands on about pregnancy loss and learning felt like therapy. Here is some of what I learned while I was trying to come to terms with my loss and figure out why it had happened: A miscarriage is the loss of a fetus before the 20th week of the pregnancy. It's more common during the 7th and 8th weeks. In the first sonogram, which is performed in the 7th or 8th week of the pregnancy, you can hear the baby's heartbeat. If everything looks normal then, the probability of miscarriage drops to 3 to 4 percent.

The risk of miscarriage increases with age, for instance, for a woman of 45 years of age, it's around 80 percent! The figures are terrifying. What I read both enlightens and scares me. In fact, when you've had two or more miscarriages, the risk is higher in subsequent pregnancies. That means, even if I conceive once again, I'm running a higher risk of miscarriage compared to those who conceive for the first time. As if it's not bad enough to have lost two...

The embryos that fail to develop properly spontaneously abort at the early stages of pregnancy, which can be regarded as an instance of natural selection, a good thing in a way, allowing the good ones to stay alive and killing off the weaker or poorly ones before they are born. We all know that when we have a miscarriage, we experience a deep sorrow and deception, a huge feeling of failure is always present. We blame ourselves. We wonder if we have done something wrong. Miscarriages may inflict women with serious emotional wounds that may be hard to heal. The most common emotions experienced after miscarriage are despair and resentment, and, of course, a deep sorrow, a kind of bereavement. Everyone has their own way of licking their wounds, but I believe having the support of our loved ones has a very soothing effect. It is very important to seek professional help to go through this period as grief may lead to depression and losing your baby when you were that close to being a mother may be devastating.

The second most common feeling after grief experienced by women who have a miscarriage is guilt. We keep blaming ourselves for what we did or didn't do while we were pregnant, for the drugs we used before pregnancy, for having had too many drinks at that party. Doctors usually don't fret about what we may have been doing before finding out we are expecting. The present and the future are more important than the past. Contrary to popular belief, a busy work life, activities such as exercising or sex, lifting heavy weights, standing for too long, reaching up to hang clothes to dry do not cause a miscarriage, whereas the risk may increase if you've had an infection during the first months of pregnancy, if you have an existing hormonal problem or a condition such as diabetes or a thyroid disease, and women with such conditions are advised to see a doctor before pregnancy to make sure all necessary precautions are taken, which all health-conscious women today would do anyway when they start preparing for pregnancy. Smoking, drinking, and doing drugs – even though they are a no-no during pregnancy – are not among direct causes of miscarriages.

Sometimes we want doctors to explain to us the reason for everything, we expect satisfactory answers, but you shouldn't expect them to give you clear-cut answers for these kind of miscarriages.

Sometimes they don't know the reason either, as it is usually the case for such miscarriages. They examine the embryo only after the third miscarriage to see if it has any genetic defects. The parents are given a series of tests and the causes are investigated. Most of the time, the tests are inconclusive, which means most pregnancy losses occur for no other reason than natural selection. If a cause is discovered, precautionary measures are taken to avoid subsequent losses.

Although this is what science tells us, I just can't be satisfied without a logical explanation. Many doctors to whom I've asked whether women had to have three miscarriages, to go through this ordeal three times, to learn about the causes, always gave me the same answer, which was it was normal or insignificant to have one or two miscarriages, and it was only after the third one that something out of the ordinary was suspected and the causes were investigated. That's just the way it is, it's the realm of the physicians and if they say it is so, there's nothing to say. It just doesn't make sense to me, but I have to accept it as a fact of life, like many other things...

Hormonal disorders rank first among the causes of miscarriages. Progesterone, the hormone that maintains the pregnancy, is secreted by the ovaries at first and by the placenta as the pregnancy proceeds and its deficiency leads to miscarriage. Progesterone deficiency can be treated by hormone replacement. Fluctuations in the levels of prolactin, known as the lactation hormone, also cause infertility and miscarriages. Also, thyroid hormone levels higher or lower than normal can lead to pregnancy losses, which can be prevented with treatment. Anomalies, that is, malformations, of the uterus can also lead to miscarriages.

Double uterus or an incompetent cervix are other causes leading to recurring miscarriages, which can be diagnosed by various imaging techniques. Cervical incompetence can be treated using cervical cerclage, which consists of making sutures at the opening of the cervix in the early stages of the pregnancy to allow it to reach its term, whereas malformations of the uterus can be surgically treated. Another possible cause of miscarriages is chromosomal disorders. If there is a family history of genetic conditions, recurring miscarriages may occur, in which case the couple should get genetic tests done and consult a specialist if an anomaly is found.

As with many other ailments, the underlying cause of recurring miscarriages can be related to our immune system, which is the defense mechanism of our body. It's thanks to our immune system that we don't usually go down with the same disease a second time; we don't have the diseases we've had as children again later in life. But there may be some problems with our immune system, which cause the mother's body to produce antibodies to some agents that normally occur in pregnancy. This, in turn, may cause recurring miscarriages. Phospholipids are one of the constituents of the body's cell structure. When the body produces anti-phospholipid antibodies, the blood flow in the placenta is compromised, resulting in coagulation and consequently, miscarriage. Women who have a miscarriage for these kind of autoimmune factors are treated with anti-coagulant drugs, the most common of which is aspirin,* which thins the blood. The treatment may even include

---

* I used both baby aspirin and anticoagulant injections during my pregnancy to prevent blood clots. Neither have any harmful side effects. The doctors in the US and Turkey use

the use of cortisone to suppress the immune system.

Never-Ending Tests

In the medical world, one miscarriage is considered as a normal instance of natural selection. The second miscarriage may be taken more seriously by some doctors, while some still consider it normal. After the third miscarriage, the situation is considered worth investigating. But neither Cosimo nor I could face dealing with a third miscarriage, we couldn't just sit still and wait until we would lose a third baby before starting to investigate the causes of our first two losses. We wanted to find out the reasons behind our two failed pregnancies. We asked around and decided to take it to the Dexeus Institute once more. The labyrinth-like floor plan had driven me mad the first time I had been in the hospital there, but in time I got used both to the hospital and to speaking Spanish and learned to find my way around. The complexity of the plan arose from the fact the building had had to be extended with the addition of new wings as the original building could not accommodate the growing institute. There was no room for further extensions, so they were soon going to move to their new, gigantesque building. What really mattered was that it was a hospital full of excellent physicians.

The tests that had to be run to determine the cause of our miscarriages involved not only me but Cosimo as well. We had

---

this method widely in the treatment of pregnant women, although it is not preferred in Europe. As a matter of fact, Turkish doctors follow the medical developments in the US closely.

to have the test results before consulting the doctors. We were ready to do whatever it took. We knew we were starting a long and daunting process, but we were trying to make the best of it, by joking and laughing about it most of the time. Although I couldn't wait for the results, I could guess what they would indicate, I expected it to be linked to the hormonal imbalance problems I'd had years ago, during puberty. I thought this was the reason why babies couldn't develop properly in my womb. I must have some hormonal deficiencies and needed hormonal supplements during pregnancy to help the fetus grow. I did trust the doctors, but I knew myself better than they ever could. In fact, I was to find out I was right about my guesses and resent the doctors' failure to do what was necessary during the early stages of my pregnancy. With a little precaution much could have been solved without any damage. Not that I didn't blame myself at all; if I hadn't been moving from one country to another and obliged to entrust myself to doctors who were not familiar with me and my medical history, obliged to start all over each time, maybe none of this would have happened. I was swinging from one extreme to the other. One day I was thinking, 'This is going to happen, I'll soon be holding my baby in my arms, as soon as the results come back we will do whatever it takes, turn over a new leaf, and this time we will make it.' The next day it was, 'There is always a problem, a setback, I will never have a baby'.

The doctors had ordered a whole bunch of tests. We were hurrying about in the labyrinth of corridors at the basement floor of the Dexeus hospital like two robots, doing what we were told. We got all the tests done; the tests for the male partner, including sperm analysis to examine the quantity and motility of the sperm, took less time. Genetic tests were required for both partners, but the ones for the female partner were somehow more comprehensive. There were all kinds of hormonal tests to see any deficiencies or excesses. I had to have an X-ray of the uterus to check for malformations, and a test to monitor ovulation.

Finally, we had all the required tests done...

What a Romantic Womb I have!

We got the results after a long and nervous waiting period. Everything looked fine. The only thing that stood out was that the top of my uterus looked a little flatter than normal – if you were to visualize the uterus as a similar shape to a heart; you could say mine was a little broader and flatter. This wasn't considered as a cause of miscarriage and wouldn't cause any trouble in pregnancy either, but the doctors advised for it to be surgically corrected. So, all in all, the reason for my miscarriages was still unknown... How romantic it was to have a womb in the shape of a heart! Mine had a flat heart shape and had to be corrected.

The team of specialists in the famous Dexeus University Hospital had met and decided my uterus had to be surgically corrected. They didn't think my previous miscarriages had anything to do with this as this malformation would only affect the pregnancy in the later stages, but they advised that it should be corrected using an endoscopic surgery technique called hysteroscopy, as a precautionary measure to avoid any problems in future pregnancies. Honestly, I didn't expect this, and I found the idea of having an operation after the recent abortion I'd just had extremely repulsive; but the promise of having a baby gave me the courage to endure any hardship. I wanted to do anything I could and to remove all the obstacles on my way, so I started to prepare for surgery without delay. I was scheduled to have it in two weeks. Well, we hadn't seen this coming, we had a trip to Andalusia planned, but were we going to be able to take it?

❦

I'm talking to Sibel on the phone and I tell her "I'm having plastic surgery on my womb."

Funny girl," says Sibel, laughing. "You would have lost your mind long ago if you didn't have this great sense of humor. Is this about having a baby again?"

Sibel was a very close friend of mine who just couldn't understand our insistence on having a baby, when it was so difficult to have and to raise one. Maybe it was because she was attached to her freedom or she hadn't met the right person, yet. Or, perhaps it was because she satisfied the thirst of her maternal instincts with the love of her beautiful, Canadian-Turkish niece, that she was not interested in having a child at all. She was very passionate about fashion and travel, two things she could never give up. We had planned to go on a tour of Andalusia; we were to meet in Seville, rent a car and drive around Andalusia for eight days.

Sevilla & Bull Fighting

We didn't cancel our trip to Andalusia. The doctors had told us that it was a minor surgery and that I only had to rest a few days and abstain from having baths for a month afterwards. I was free to go on with my life as usual. My dearest mother, as soon as she had heard the word 'surgery,' had jumped on a plane and come to Barcelona to be near me. I'd been asked to report to the hospital early in the morning on the day of the surgery, but the operation didn't take place until late afternoon. It was very annoying to have to wait in a hospital room in an operation gown for the hours to pass. Having rested for a few days after surgery, I was cleared by my doctor to go on the trip and we left for Seville, with my mother with us. It was March, a lovely month to see the south of Spain. The temperature often exceeds 40 degrees Celsius in Andalusia in July and August, forcing not only people but all living things to stay inside during the day time, and go out and live at night. So, it wouldn't be a good time to travel around.

The climate of Andalusia resembles that of the countries in North Africa, the influences of which can also be seen on the culture, a magnificent example being the Alhambra Palace, a must-see for all tourists. We had bought our tickets on the Internet well in advance, and booked our hotels. When you travel to a country, like Spain, which attracts millions of tourists every year, you have to plan your trip very carefully. Otherwise, you may have to pay exorbitant prices to stay in humble hotel rooms and stand in queues for hours under the sun to enter museums. Our trip was going very well, we were all in good spirits, and nothing went wrong except for the battery of the car we'd rented in Malaga, the city of Picasso, dying. How beautiful everything was! Andalusia was a splendid region with its landscapes, architecture, people and cuisine. The only thing that put a damper on the trip was me constantly worrying about my operation wounds. I felt very limited by my fears of over-exerting myself. Everything would have been much better if I could just let go...

The Bathtub Adventure in the Hotel Room

I will never forget the moment when I jumped out of the bathtub...
We were all exhausted at the end of a day where we had walked
the streets of Seville inch by inch. We retired to our rooms to
rest a while before dinner. Cosimo was so tired he fell asleep as
soon as he lay down on the bed. I thought I would rest my legs
and my soul with a nice warm bath. I turned the bathroom into a
spa instantly, lighting the little scented candles I always carry in
my toiletry bag, filled the tub and poured in all the shower gels I
could find and sank in the bubbly water. But... it occurred to me
all of sudden that I'd just had surgery a week ago and I wasn't
meant to have a bath for a month, to prevent any infections! I
had totally forgotten about it and sunk in the hot water with my
stitches. I couldn't believe just how quickly I jumped out of the
water. How careless of me! I was mad at myself. Not only was my
spa session interrupted, but now, I had to obsess over whether I
had hurt my wound during the five minutes I'd spent in the tub.
It was a good thing we were on holiday, with so much around –
castanets, mantillas, Flamenco, Sevillana,* bull fights, sun and sea,
seafood, wine, and more wine – to distract me. But, being who I
am, I couldn't keep myself from feeling guilty. Not even admiring
our favorite matador with Sibel could make me forget the incident
of the hot bath for one moment...

Back to Trying to Having a Baby After the Trip

Now that even the slightest obstacles were removed from our

---

* A type of music and dance of Seville, Spain.

way, we thought we would start trying again straight away. Some friends had suggested we see Dr. Leila Onbargi, an American ob-gyn, whom we had contacted to get an appointment. She greeted us with a welcoming smile. I love doctors like this, who convey positive energy to their patients. You know, if you are going to see a doctor, you must have a certain problem, you are worried and distressed. You don't want to see a sulky, grim face, do you?

So, anyway, I tell her my whole medical history. She takes notes, asks me the name and dosage of the ovary-stimulating hormone pills I used to take. I have a health folder that I take to every doctor's appointment with me that keeps growing thicker, so I'm able to answer all her questions immediately and clearly. "You've come prepared," she says. Well, I have to be, considering I go from one doctor to another, from one country to another... She prescribes a pill with a lower dose than the ones I used in Turkey, "because I think this is as much as you need," she says, and tells me I should start using it on the fifth day of my period if I feel ready to get pregnant. She wishes us good luck and we thank her and leave with fresh hopes...

Oh, No! I Have My Period!

I woke up that morning with pain in my pelvis. I had had an uncomfortable night because of intermittent pains that kept waking me up and I felt tired. I went straight to the bathroom (as I always do when I get up) and saw that I had my period. How disheartening it was! It was eight months since we'd been trying and we hadn't got there yet. My doctor had prescribed an injection drug to help the release of eggs from the ovary in addition to the ovary-stimulating pills I was using. I had been going to the doctor's office every month during my ovulation period, so I could be given a shot when the eggs had matured. It was crucial that the partners have intercourse during the 36-hour window following the injection. Having to have sex within a certain period of time turned it into some kind of task. You couldn't be the same person every day of your life, some days you might be tired or sick, some days you might be busy or feeling out of sorts. But that was the rule, you either acted on it or you were out of the game, and had to wait another month to do it all over again. I think we had tried the combination of hormone pills and injections two or three times by then, to no avail.

Will we now have to deal with infertility, as well? As if miscarriages weren't enough! In my two previous pregnancies, I managed to conceive in the same month when I started to take the little white pills. I'm now annoyed by and impatient with the therapy, which doesn't work. 'Working' at making a baby during given days every month is stressful. Sex has become a task to be fulfilled, a drag. This brings me down. I'm worried that we could be ruining our relationship trying to complete it with a baby. Fortunately, I'm a very positive person and my husband is a very compassionate and sensible man. He looks quite relaxed and calm, probably because he loves me and really wants to have a child. I marvel that love makes you endure so much; if we can bear all this to have a child; God knows what we could stand when we have one.

I do a quick Internet search, and find out that a couple may be considered infertile if they haven't been able to conceive after one year of regular sexual intercourse, in which case they are advised to get medical help without delay. The male partner has to be tested first, as the tests for the female partner are more tedious and take longer, of course, that's a woman's lot! We always get the tough part of everything! The most common problems causing infertility in women are endometriosis (benign cysts), ovulation disorders, low egg quality, blocked fallopian tubes and, uterine and vaginal anomalies, whereas in men the most widespread causes are sperm problems such as low sperm count or malformed sperm, or blockage of sperm transport. In approximately 15 to 20 percent of couples there is no obvious underlying cause and this is classified as 'unexplained infertility'.

We had already got all these tests done, so we had the results. My uterus was slightly out of shape, which was corrected by a surgery, so we seemed to fall into this last category of 'unexplained infertility'. Everything that was happening to us felt like a cruel joke. I couldn't help asking myself why I had to be part of the minority instead of the majority. I admit I've always felt different, but at that moment I felt I could give up so much just to be an ordinary woman. The more I read, the more depressed I felt.

I called my husband and we decided to meet for lunch. It did me good to chat with him over lunch, he cheered me up. After I dropped him back off at work I went window shopping in Avenue Diagonal, one of the loveliest avenues in Barcelona where you could find the most stylish stores. Window shopping was refreshing, I loved it. You didn't need to try anything on, or spend any money, you just had to look at the apparel on the window and visualize it on you! Even if I came across something I liked, I had no intention of trying anything on with my bulging tummy after the fine meal I'd just had. It was early spring but the windows were already full of summery clothes, the mannequins in the window were all clad in bright, cheerful colors. Suddenly, I felt lively and excited. I told myself, like the famous line from that Cem Yılmaz movie, "Everything's gonna be great!"

❦

We made up our mind; we don't want to keep trying for months on end and lose any more time. We go to see Dr. Leila again, who tells us there is apparently nothing wrong with us and suggests artificial insemination. "It's the first method we advise our patients to try, and in case this doesn't work, the second step to take is to try in vitro fertilization," she says. The concept of artificial insemination goes as far back as humanity but it began to be used in livestock in its modern sense in early 20th century. For a moment, I think of cows: My father bred cattle for some years besides farming, when I was a young child. I remember the vet coming to the farm to inseminate the cows. It turns out this old technique can now be applied to humans. You don't hear of such things unless you need them.

As the doctor tells us about the procedure, I smile as I remember the depressed cows... Once we were staying in a hotel in the midst of a cattle farm in Costa Brava, the Catalans' famous holiday resort. Although there were a good many pregnant cows and calves on the farm, which used to sell their milk to the Danone Company, the bulls were nowhere to be seen, which made us wonder how the cows bred. When we put the question to the landlady over coffee after breakfast, she told us that breeding was done through artificial insemination and therefore keeping bulls was unnecessary. Obviously the Spanish didn't want their bulls to waste their energy on breeding. The cows lived away from the bulls, they didn't look too cheerful; they looked rather depressed. Well, it was a new world where you didn't need a male partner to get pregnant and the cows just followed the trend, but they had to live alone, a life without sex. Every time I have a cup of Danone yogurt, I remember the depressed cows and smile...

Although it sounds like good news that everything looks fine, we obviously do have a problem stopping us from having a baby. What are we to do now? Our doctor advises us to consult an infertility center without delay, before I get older. It looks like the right thing to do. Barcelona has a number of very good infertility centers, so renowned in fact that people come from overseas to realize their dreams of having a baby. But it would complicate things for us to start this move here in Barcelona, because we will soon be relocating again, this time to Brussels. Frankly, I don't feel like moving at all, I love Barcelona, where we've been living for two full years. But I resist the temptation of getting attached to it, because Barcelona is a tempting city, like Javier Bardem,* my favorite Spanish actor...

I don't wish to make the same mistake I made when I was moving here from Istanbul, but I don't wish to wait too long

---

* The Spanish have a kind of fried potatoes they call 'patatas bravas', where the potatoes are chopped into irregular chunks, oil fried, and covered with ground red pepper. Javier Bardem reminds me of those, he is not one of those neat, baby-faced actors, he looks rather untidy, even sloppy, but he is hot, delicious and irresistibly charismatic!

and be late, either. Back there, in Istanbul, I had put off getting pregnant for two years with the concern that we might move at any time, but the relocation we expected took longer than we'd thought to realize and two years went by waiting for the news. If I had a chance to go back in time, I would start trying to conceive straight away, while I was still young, without thinking about Cosimo's work situation, the relocation, the moving, or anything else. But back then I wasn't in a hurry to have a baby and I felt more concerned about the move, I'd recently had a miscarriage, I was sad and disheartened, I was expecting a great change in my life which I had to prepare for, I was going to leave my country and go overseas... When I thought of all the concerns related to pregnancy, I didn't dare shouldering such a burden. That was how I felt then, so I'd decided to postpone having a baby for a while.

But now, it's different. I'm both ready and determined. As soon as we go to Brussels, I'm going to find the doctor in that infertility center that Dr. Leila told me about. We are turning the Barcelona page over and heading towards a new life in Brussels...

3

Brussels

It was our second year in Barcelona. Cosimo came home from work one night with an envelope in his hand and asked me to pick a city: "Where would you like to go?" he said, "Rome, or Paris, or Brussels?" The envelope contained a complimentary flight ticket for two from Alitalia Airlines that we fly regularly. We got to choose from three cities. We'd both been to Rome and Paris several times while we'd never been to Brussels. I'd been following the fashion and furniture design news from Belgium and admiring the works of young, avant-garde designers. "Let's go to Brussels, then," I said, to which Cosimo agreed and we flew to Brussels for an extended weekend before Christmas.

Brussels was a city with a little Mediterranean spirit added to a northern life style. It pleased us as soon as we saw it. We went all around it by tram during our 4-day stay, leaving no side street unseen. We wondered at the ethnic variety we saw on the streets, where most of the grocer's stores were owned and run by Asian, Middle Eastern or South African families, with all the family members working in the shop. These people lived in Brussels without changing their habits from back home, in their traditional apparel. I thought its people from various ethnic origins were adding color to an otherwise grey Brussels, which had given me the impression of a small-scale London with its rainy, foggy, overcast sky and constant humidity; it looked like London's little brother.

Since I love London, I warmed to it quickly and said to Cosimo, "I could live in this city," without suspecting even so slightly that in two months' time Cosimo would come to me to tell he'd been contacted by the bank manager to let him know he was needed in the bank's Brussels office and that we were relocate in less than three months! In Turkey, in such situations we say "I could have thought of something else instead and it would have come true!" When Cosimo told me of the relocation and asked me how I felt about it, at I first hesitated, because we hadn't had our fill of Barcelona,* we'd only been here for two years and it was ideal for my career, my business was starting to liven up, my circle of friends to grow larger. But even if we decided to decline and stay here, the bank was bound to come with another offer, sooner than later, and we might be faced with relocating to another city which we might not like. So, we felt compelled to say yes to Brussels, but we didn't feel inconvenienced. The Brussels episode of our adventure began

---

* Barcelona may be one of the greatest cities to live in, but every rose has its thorn. You always feel like a foreigner in Barcelona, you live a foreigner's life and don't really mingle with the Catalans. If there are any Catalans you get to know closely they are sure to have lived outside of Catalonia sometime in their life or to be married to a foreigner, otherwise they are too conservative to go around with foreigners, or even Spanish people from other parts of the country. A friend of mine from Madrid once said, "If you were to live here a hundred years, the Catalans would always reject you and make you feel an alien. I, for one, feel that way even though I'm Spanish, how could you not?"

in the summer of 2005...

Although we regretted leaving Barcelona for Brussels, the capital of Europe endeared itself to us quickly. Our amiable landlord Jean Pierre was quite a character, renowned for his honesty in Brussels. Although he did make us suffer, we have to admit that he was very supportive and helpful in every way he could have been. We adapted quite quickly as we didn't experience any problems in communicating with people. Everybody spoke English as it was the second language used by the Flemish. Because we used English in every aspect of our daily lives, we were rather slow in learning French. It became important for me to enroll in a class as well as make some friends who only spoke French. We were getting used to our new home and to life in Brussels. Now it was time to take up our dream of having a baby, we had to take action without delay.

We called Dr. Camus, the physician in chief of the infertility center at the university hospital, whom Dr. Leila, my ob-gyn from back in Barcelona, had recommended. The earliest appointment date available was in a month, as it is usually the case with the doctors in European hospitals, you cannot normally get an appointment within a shorter time period than a month unless you have an emergency. I'm still not sure I understand the reason for this but I think this is due to the appointments accumulating because of limited working hours. So we waited for a month before finally going to the Academische Ziekenhuis Vrije Universiteit Brussels (AZ-VUB) Hospital.

First Insemination

We are in Dr. Camus' office. At first I go over my medical history down to the last detail, as have done so many times before, I know it by heart now, the sentences just flow effortlessly. Then I answer the doctor's questions. When I'm finished, Dr. Camus states that we are going to use the artificial insemination technique, which is the first step of assisted reproductive technology (ART). I explain that I got pregnant twice before, using hormone supplements but without recourse to ART, and ask the probable reason why it's just not happening this time. Dr. Camus, choosing his words carefully like most doctors, tells me that ovulation rate decreases as a woman's age advances and adds, "When a couple doesn't succeed in getting pregnant naturally in over a year, it would be best to start treatment without waiting further."

To think that I believed I could get pregnant just by swallowing a tiny pill! I thought my only problem was not being able to stay pregnant, I didn't expect to be unable to get pregnant in the first place. Things are getting tangled and I'm growing worried. My mother was highly fecund; she got pregnant many times by accident. When my parents wanted to have me, she got pregnant as soon as the first month, and the same with my brother. She never had a miscarriage. It's obvious I don't take after my mother! My paternal aunt was married three times but didn't have any children. I wonder if it's after her that I take? Will I remain childless like her?

My mind wandering off to these thoughts has distracted me from what the doctor's saying. I focus, and hear him say the following: "When a couple has difficulty having a baby or they cannot get pregnant after a year of sexual intercourse without contraception, there may be a question of infertility. As long as there are no other underlying causes, for young couples like you who cannot conceive naturally when there is no obvious explanation, we start with applying artificial insemination as a first step of treatment." That's nice! The doctor's just called us a young couple. The doctor goes on: "In this center, we repeat the treatment up to three times. Not that there are any problems associated with further applications, but it is statistically meaningless. If this method doesn't work, then we will proceed to the next step without delay, which is in vitro fertilization (IVF)."

We make up our minds: We tell the doctor we want to start the treatment. He calls a young midwife into the office, "This is my assistant, Ilse Diricks," he says. "She will explain the details of the treatment. Good luck, see you later." So the treatment starts. In truth, our doctor only appears as a name on our file, we never see him again after the first appointment. From then on we just follow the routine. Ilse, the specialist nurse to take care of us, has us fill out some forms and asks us dozens of questions as she wants to make sure that we have had all the necessary tests and exams done. Then she briefs us about the procedure, which is not all that complicated. I have to go to the hospital every other day following the 12th day of my cycle to do an ultrasound following my ovulation period. When the eggs are the adequate size, I'll be given a shot to stimulate their release, followed by the insemination, which consists of placing the sperm collected from the male partner into the vagina through a plastic tube (catheter). The procedure doesn't take longer than 15 minutes and the sperm is released into the female reproductive system. Of course, there will be some preparations before the procedure, which our nurse will tell us about when the time comes.

All we have to do now is to wait for my next period and then call the hospital to start the hormone injections. I am now registered in the control center of the hospital, called Monitor. They have all my personal information and the details of my treatment schedule, and their job is to remind me of all the things I have to do daily and to oversee my treatment. We start on our adventure. The day we've been expecting comes and the show is on. I am very excited, this is the first time I'll have the injection. My husband is there with me, to share moment. I have the shot and pray everything goes smoothly.

I have no idea about the dosage of hormone I'm given, I have to trust the specialists and their competency. They know all about my medical story, the drugs I have taken so far and their effects on me. These hormone injections are meant to stimulate my lazy ovaries. After the shots, I start to receive the calls from the Monitor to go to the hospital every other day following the 12th day of my cycle to follow the growth of the follicles through ultrasound.

It's eight in the morning. I'm reading a leaflet about artificial insemination in the waiting room of the infertility center. We are waiting our turn like everybody else. We hear our name being called, Cosimo is ushered to a small room and handed a plastic laboratory cup. What he has to do is obvious; he needs to collect his sperm in the cup and hand it to the lab. It's quite repulsive and weird but it's the only way to go, take it or leave it! Men having to collect sperm in a plastic cup is nothing compared to the innumerable repulsive or weird procedures that women have to undergo; we have to carry all the burden, like always. Everything takes place in our body. Being a mother is the hardest, toughest job on earth, and men are there to support us. Well, we have to give them credit for putting up with us when our hormones go crazy...

I keep refreshing my knowledge about AI. I've studied every step so well I know everything by heart now, but I still read the leaflet with interest, to pass the time waiting for Cosimo. There are some requirements for a successful insemination, the first of which is the presence of an egg to be fertilized, that is, it won't work if you have a problem with your ovulation. If your ovaries are lazy (as is the case with me), ovulation is stimulated with hormone supplements, as a first step, followed by hormone injections to stimulate the release of the eggs. The second requirement is that the tubes must be in a condition to allow the sperm to reach the egg. It must be seen on the X-ray that they are open. Then, the male partner's sperm analysis results must be normal or at least close to normal, AI won't work for people who have no or too little sperm. Finally, no endometrial pathology (which means no wounds on the uterine lining) must be present that could prevent the fertilized egg from attaching to the uterine wall. AI is used most commonly in situations where the sperm motility is low (when the sperm are lazy) or when the cervical secretions of the female partner do not allow the sperm to move properly – well, I've heard of women rejecting men before, but this is the first time I've heard of women rejecting men's sperm!

The advantage of AI over natural sexual intercourse is that it overcomes the cervical factor and shortens the distance the sperm must cover. The male partner must abstain from sexual intercourse for three days before the procedure, which our doctor emphatically repeated a few times. On the day of the procedure, the male partner collects and gives his sperm. The preferred method for the collection of sperm is masturbation, where no lubricating oils or gels are allowed as they may interfere with the quality of sperm. The semen sample obtained is processed with certain chemicals.

Then, the female partner lies down in the gynecological exam position and a speculum is inserted. The cervix is washed with saline solution, a catheter is inserted all the way into the uterine cavity and the sperm is placed in the uterus, after which the catheter and the speculum are removed. It's normal that some sperm comes out. AI is not a painful procedure. After the procedure the patient has to lie down for 10 to 15 minutes, after which she can resume her normal life.

As an option, the patient may be given progesterone supplements. She is advised to abstain from heavy physical activity for the first 24 to 48 hours after the procedure, but she doesn't need to stay in bed. If she doesn't get her period in two weeks from the procedure, a pregnancy test is done. If it comes out positive, prenatal care is started. If it comes negative, the patient is called in for an ultrasound on the third day of her period to start a new cycle of AI. The success rate is about 5 to 20 percent, the chances increase with increasing number of tries. Theoretically, there is no harm in continuing to try but it is not advised that you should go on trying after 6 or 7 failed attempts, as normally three attempts should be all you need if AI works for you.

Passengers in a Plastic Cup

Cosimo finally emerges from the room. He looks self-conscious. Everyone in the waiting room knows what the men coming out of the small rooms are carrying in the little plastic cups. This can obviously be quite embarrassing. They should have taken the patients' sensibility into consideration and built these rooms a little further out of sight. I immediately start designing a new hospital in my mind, starting with the gynecologic exam rooms, which have to be changed from top to bottom, especially the patients' changing rooms... Women have a very fussy eye, especially when you are an architect like me you can't help seeing all the details and look for perfection and beauty everywhere.

Cosimo teases me, saying, "What if they mixed up the cups in the lab and you gave birth to an Asian baby?"* This may only be a joke but I'm sure such mistakes do happen, there is the human factor to consider, and even machines can make mistakes... Patients in the waiting room can't help but to peer at the people who go in

---

* During our frequent visits to the hospital, we started to recognize some of the other couples like us coming for treatment. Observing the other patients and seeing different people was the most entertaining part of being in the hospital. Many of the hospitals in Europe are Catholic hospitals run by nuns. AZ-VUB Hospital was different as it was a 'secular' university hospital, open to people from all religious backgrounds, and hence was flooded with people from all over Europe (especially from countries like Italy where there are restrictions on IVF treatment because of the Vatican's influence) coming in for treatment. All these people from different races, religions and cultures, speaking different languages, and wearing different clothing, had one thing in common, one thing that brought them here: THE DESIRE TO HAVE A BABY.

and out of the small room. Cosimo and I keep commenting about them. I know it's not nice but we have to distract ourselves and this is the most innocent distraction at hand, it doesn't hurt anyone. We hear our name being called and end our fantasy of different baby combinations. You have to make fun of these situations.

We go into the exam room, where a nurse meets us at the door. Her hands are full of tubes, syringes and different instruments. I lie down on the exam table, in pelvic exam position, where I wait for the insemination. Another nurse comes from the lab carrying a tube full of sperm.* They proceed with what they have to do without any explanation. I don't feel much except the typical sensation of cold and stretching when the speculum is inserted. The cold saline solution they use to wash the vagina makes me shiver. I also shiver from agitation, which adds to the feeling of

---

* Society today sees a change in the concept of family. It no longer takes a man and a woman, bound in matrimony, to have a child, in fact, a man is not needed at all. A single woman, or two women – a homosexual couple, married or living together – can apply to an infertility center. All they need is the sperm from a man, which can be obtained from a sperm bank, a fertility clinic or a donor they know, then artificial insemination is performed and a baby is born with two mothers. Or, a single man wishing to have a baby can have his wish come true today, using a surrogate mother willing to 'lend their womb for the duration of a pregnancy. (In the USA, Hollywood stars who do not wish to be pregnant commonly resort to surrogate mothers.) Then the father-to-be can have a baby with the surrogate mother or another woman he chooses with in vitro fertilization. Children with two mothers grow up without a father, and those with two fathers without a mother. It seems difficult to accept it when in some families, both parents are of the same sex. It might even feel strange to think of it, but the world is changing whether we like it or not and it's up to you to either go with it or stay behind.

cold. My dear husband is right beside me! He is just as nervous as I am, watching everything that's going on. And, it's done! The sperm are placed where they should be. Now all we have to do is pray that they find the right eggs and fertilize them.

❦

Insemination takes only about 10 minutes. I'm advised to rest for another 10 minutes on the exam table, in half-lying position. I play it safe and don't move for at least 20 minutes, until the nurses have to almost kick me out, saying it's another patient's turn. I get up reluctantly, hoping the passengers have reached their destination. I hang on Cosimo's arm as we walk to our car in the hospital's parking lot, with slow steps as if were walking on the moon. I know it's ridiculous but sometimes you just can't bring yourself to reason. I can't wait to go home and get in bed. I try and spend a few quiet days and go back to my life as usual.

I'm to go to the laboratory of the hospital for a blood test in two weeks. The days seemed to drag on, I'm constantly thinking about whether I'm pregnant or not. What if I am? Then I should be careful. Or, is it going to end with a miscarriage again? Like every woman who has recurring miscarriages, this has become a phobia for me. I want to share my concerns with the doctor and get some satisfactory answers, but the doctor is unlikely to help me at this stage, because he treats all his expecting patients the same until a problem comes up.

I go to the lab at the third floor of the hospital where I've been coming so frequently lately to have my hormone shots, and give a blood sample. The next day, I receive a call from the Monitor:

"Congratulations, the results are positive, you are pregnant!" I cannot believe it! What I've been praying for such a long time has finally come true, I am pregnant! My voice shakes, my legs feel like water. It's like as if I'm Nur the student before an exam – the last time I remember having had such emotions is when I was 17 and about to take the admissions exam to get into university. I felt just as I do now, I felt so cold inside with anxiety that I trembled like a leaf. The very first thing I do is call my husband. "I AM PREGNANT!" Now it's his voice that's shaking when he exclaims "Great news!" He comes home early and holds me as if he never wants to let go, we stay like that, locked in an embrace, he strokes my hair while I keep trembling. I just can't get warm. There's no way I could describe my feelings at that moment.

Four Black Dots

It's our seventh week and our first prenatal appointment... We are very excited! We are going to hear that heartbeat, see that little black dot the size of a lentil. It's a different specialist who takes care of you each time you go for an ultrasound in this giant university hospital, you don't have a regular physician during the first stage of your pregnancy. The Monitor center calls you to let you know of the date of your exam. When it's your turn, you have to get undressed in one of the cubicles in a row, each narrower than the fitting rooms in stores, inside which there is nothing but a chair. You are expected to remove all your clothes below the waist the ultrasound is done through the vagina during the first trimester.

Don't bother looking around for disposable slippers or an exam gown or even a cloth to wrap around your waist like you would expect to find in Turkey, because it's not customary here to cover yourself in the exam room. Everything is extremely minimalistic, extremely cold and cost-effective! When your name is called, you come out of the changing cubicle, naked below the waist, stepping barefoot on the cold floor; you pass in front of the ultrasound specialist and his assistant that you have never seen before and lie down on the exam table. I was very embarrassed about being half naked, without so much as a wrap to cover myself, when I had my first Ob-gyn visit outside of Turkey, in Barcelona, but I've grown used to it in time and even developed my own solutions, like wearing a skirt and pulling it up when I lie down on the exam table. But here it's even worse. I and three other women like me are waiting, undressed, in the cubicles standing side by side, like race horses in the starting stalls. When your turn comes, you go into the exam room from the door on the opposite side of the cubicle to the one you came in, and after the exam you go back in the cubicle to get dressed and leave from the door you came in. In time, I got used to this as well, but at the beginning I used to find it humiliating and resented this system that I found excessively cold. Everything was extremely organized but not humane. The decrease in the amount of services provided, this 'self-service' system, was supposed to be an indicator of the level of civilization, but sometimes I find it hard to tell what is civilized and what is not.

I'm lying on the exam table in the imaging room, looking for the dark patch indicating the amniotic sac on the monochrome screen. I'm suddenly startled with a sight I cannot believe is true: There are... four sacs, meaning four embryos in my uterus! I am pregnant but I'm so shocked I cannot even rejoice. I can't take my eyes of the four dark patches. I'm totally confused; thoughts and concerns swarm in my brain. My husband is also stunned, speechless. We are just staring at the screen, focusing on what the specialist has to say, who is in turn very quiet for a while (probably because of surprise) and just keeps examining the contents of the uterus carefully, moving the probe. Yes, there are four sacs but only three of the embryos are alive. I am pregnant with triplets. A fourth egg was fertilized, the embryo was formed, but it couldn't make it.

Doctors in Europe are ill-disposed towards multiple pregnancies beyond twins. They accept twins but when there are more embryos, they terminate the weaker ones, allowing only the two that are larger and stronger. As dreadful as it sounds to a mother, you have to think of it as a precaution taken to ensure the health and well-being of the mother and of the survival of the selected embryos, and not dwell on it. I've read that in South America (especially in Mexico) they see no harm in keeping triplets, quadruplets, quintuplets, and even sextuplets in multiple pregnancies that occur naturally or as a result of assisted reproductive technology, but this is not the case in European countries.

The human uterus is fit to accommodate a single embryo, which makes multiple pregnancies a health hazard for the mother and the babies. I remember Cosimo and me hugging each other tight after coming out of the exam room, as if telling one another to be strong. We were happy, our dream was about to come true, but care and apprehension seemed to suppress our joy. How could I carry to term a multiple pregnancy when I wasn't able to do a single one? I had just about recovered from my miscarriages and decided to try again without delay. I knew the risk of miscarriage increased in multiple pregnancies, which worried me. How was I going to make it? I was scared, terrorized.

But I was also furious! I resented the hospital and the doctors in charge of my treatment, because I could remember clearly what I was told during my last ultrasound before insemination. They said there were many eggs of adequate size for fertilization. That meant there was a high probability of multiple pregnancies. I couldn't see how they could go on with the insemination when there were so many eggs. What negligence, what recklessness! They must have overdone the dose of hormonal supplements. And I had warned them time and again, telling them I had lazy ovaries but could get pregnant with minimal support. I told them everything about my past pregnancies, to the last detail. I felt infertility centers traded off better judgment in exchange for a higher success rate. They were supposed to suspend treatment in case of 'ovarian hyper stimulation syndrome.' How could they have overlooked this important detail during the ultrasound? So, what were we to do now? Were the babies and I to pay for their negligence?

Farewell to Number Three...

After the first trimester, the infertility center sends you on your way, saying, "Our job ends here, we completed our task. You are now pregnant!" Their job is helping you make babies, not deliver them. After this point you have the option of staying with the same hospital and selecting one of their ob-gyn specialists or going to a different hospital for your prenatal care. My case was different from other expecting mothers. The hospital's task, unlike the fertility center's, was not completed yet as I carried three embryos. There were more procedures to be carried out to ensure a healthy pregnancy and healthy babies. We were transferred to the hospital's department taking care of this type of special pregnancies. Dr. De Catte was an expert in this area. He examined me before the end of the first trimester.

We had to undergo a procedure called 'embryo reduction,' which meant the elimination of one of the three embryos. One of the embryos was to be selected for termination. It was one thing to expect twins, but expecting triplets entailed great risks for both the mother and the babies. A test was to be performed before the reduction, called chorionic villus sampling, or CVS,* to see whether all the embryos were well. This test was preferred because it was the earliest diagnostic tool that could be used in a pregnancy. Unlike amniocentesis, where a sample of the amniotic fluid is taken for the test, a small tissue sample is taken from the placenta for CVS. When I asked why we couldn't do an amniocentesis like everybody else, I was told succinctly that it was possible to get results sooner with CVS, and we needed a quick result as we couldn't defer reduction to wait for the embryos to grow. I was having to take such important decisions hastily, without having a chance of thinking it over. It didn't look like I had much of a choice, I had to rely on the doctors' experience and advice. So we went over the AZ-VUB Hospital on the 11th week of my pregnancy to have CVS procedure done.

---

* I found out later that CVS is twice as likely to cause a miscarriage as with amniocentesis on average and three times for triplets; it may also cause deformation of the limbs. It's a good thing I didn't know it then as I would have been 10 times more worried!

I can see all three of them clearly on the screen. I have three babies in my womb! How can I sacrifice one of them! Lord, give me strength and patience. What an ordeal! I'm scared already. I try not to keep thinking about it but I can't keep it off my mind. It's going to be hard to endure this process... I'm lying on my back on a gurney, with my hands clasped over my chest, feeling my heartbeat. I don't know whether I'm holding my hands like this in prayer or because it gives me some sort of strength, but it definitely does me good to feel myself, to listen to my own breathing. Dr. De Catte tells me to decide whether I'll keep my hands there through the procedure, because I won't be able to move them, I have to keep very still. "It's a very delicate procedure," he says. "Yes," I answer, "I'll keep them here."

My abdomen is locally anaesthetized and they prick my belly with a needle longer than a knitting needle as I watch. All I feel is like being pricked with a little pin. There is no pain but it's horrifying to look at, I cannot go on watching it, I fix my eyes on the ceiling. How can I watch myself being stabbed in the belly when I cannot even see blood? I can't even think of it! The doctor carefully inserts these long needles into my womb and takes a tissue sample from each of the placentas, while I stare at a fixed point on the ceiling, almost too scared to breathe lest I move...

The test is over. I felt next to no pain, my only concern is for the babies to be well. Tissue samples have been taken from all three placentas and are going to be examined. We have to wait for the results before the next procedure. I feel like a test subject. Fortunately, I have Cosimo with me. He grabs my hand with both hands, "I know it's hard," he says, "Hang in there, my love!" The procedure takes only 10 minutes. I'm taken on a wheelchair from the exam room to another room. I'm told to rest. I lie on the gurney for about an hour.

The doctor tells me to stay at home and rest for about a week. I have the feeling I am continuously at rest all the time. I'm an active city girl, I'm used to keeping on the move, I work, and I love to stroll along the avenues. I walk the city with a long, quick pace... When I'm at home, I don't sit for a minute, I always have something to do, even if I don't, I find something. It's not normal for me to sit down and rest, I normally rest by exercising. How drastically a baby can change a mother's life, even before it's born... I didn't believe people when they said "Your life will change when you have a baby." Now I see my life change even before I have a baby! It even changes your personality; you turn into the epitome of patience. I'm amazed at myself that I can just lay on the couch at home without complaining...

The Embryo Reduction

They call it "reduction." It's just a euphemism for extermination... "Reduction," they say! They inject potassium into the embryo's little heart and its life of 12 weeks comes to an end; a quick procedure...

We find out from the tests that all three embryos are totally healthy... which makes it even harder. Which one is to go? Which one of the triplets shall we choose to sacrifice? The doctor says it's best to pick the smallest in such circumstances as the bigger ones are also stronger. He asks us whether we approve of his decision so he can fill out his paperwork. We reply we are there because we trust his judgment. And the procedure begins. This time only one needle is inserted through my belly as the target in known. To be honest, I feel nothing at the moment of reduction. I do feel a certain sadness after I leave the hospital but I find solace in thinking that the other two are healthy... What I feel is similar to the feelings of a mother who, although she is devastated by the loss of a child, is grateful for her other children's being well, and strives to survive and be strong for them. Again, I have to stay at home and rest for a week. I find it rather hard to endure and I spend my days praying for the twins to stay safe and sound.

The Risky First Trimester is Over

I am through my 12th week, I'm overjoyed. Today we have a sonogram scheduled with Dr. De Catte at the hospital. The twins seem to be growing just fine; I am now a normal pregnant woman who has only routine prenatal visits to go to. This department of the hospital takes care of critical pregnancies only. Dr. De Catte and I say goodbye to each other because I will be going to another hospital closer to where I live from now on and he will be transferring to another hospital as well. He's been offered a position of chief physician in the infertility ward of another important university hospital in Belgium. With my doctor gone, there will be nothing holding me in AZ-VUB hospital, which is quite a distance from our home. We live in the south of Brussels, while the hospital is in the north. Furthermore, we have to drive through a tunnel of 15-20 kilometers long that crosses the city from end to end. What if there is a traffic jam in the tunnel while we are driving to the hospital for labor? You cannot just get out of the tunnel so quickly. I may be becoming overly anxious, dwelling on my worst fears, but I don't like taking risks, I feel I'd be more comfortable with a hospital that we can reach more easily.

We have been in Brussels for five months. Our network of friends is expanding thanks to Cosimo's business relationships and my social skills, and we are getting used to our new city. There are quite a number of Turkish people living in Brussels and I don't feel so lonely. From time to time, when I feel a longing for Turkey, I go to the Turkish quarter with its Turkish grocers, markets, butchers, and even jewelers, kebab and 'lahmacun' restaurants. Just the smell of the air there cheers me up.

Brussels has two languages, with French as the majority language. I don't feel comfortable if I don't understand the conversations of people on the street, the TV, the newspapers in a place where I live. I decide to take a French class. I wouldn't be able to take up a job while I am expecting twins anyway, so I go back to being a student, as it looks like the best thing to do. I have class for four hours every morning, learning French, I am drowning in grammar! I become friendly with my classmates very quickly. Together we make up a small, multinational group befitting of Brussels, people from Ghana, India, Japan, Norway, Sweden, Turkey, Poland, Vietnam, Czechoslovakia; you name it. After school we go out for lunch together, unfortunately we speak English among ourselves, so where, and when, am I supposed to practice my French, I don't know. Our French teacher Carmen is a Frenchwoman from Spanish origin, "Don't get your hopes too high," she says, "this is not France. The French will refuse to talk English even if they know it, but the Belgian people love speaking to you in English." She tells us she still feels like a stranger here even though she's been living here for 30 years. French is an extremely strange language anyway, we bend over backwards to pronounce eight vowels in a row. Besides, knowing just French won't do, you have to speak Dutch as well to get a job.

I meet a young Norwegian man in our class who happens to be married and whose wife is seven months pregnant. He tells me that they are perfectly satisfied with the doctor who oversees their pregnancy and that the ladies in the European Commission favor him too. Furthermore, the Edith Cavell hospital where she works is among the oldest and most reliable hospitals in Brussels, or even in Belgium, renowned for their ob-gyn center. A Belgian friend of mine who is 60 years old tells me he was born there and that the Edith Cavell was one of the best even then. And...it's only five minutes from where we live! How lucky is that! So, thanks to my desire of avoiding a stressful trip on my way to the hospital that I meet Dr. Markowich. I call her straight away to schedule our first appointment.

Although she delivers at the Edith Cavell, Dr. Markowich's office is somewhere else. In Brussels, physicians from different branches join together to form 'Health Centers,' as we have lately started to see similar enterprises in Istanbul, I'm familiar with the concept. My first appointment with Dr. Markowich takes about an hour and a half. She keeps typing away as she records the information about my medical history, which is rather complicated, onto her computer. She listens attentively and takes notes. We communicated easily as her English is very fluent and she is a woman. I have to see another doctor every month for the ultrasounds, which I find a little strange and annoying. I have to pay Dr. Markowich just to talk to her, she won't examine me, and I have to come back in 15 days after the ultrasound to discuss it. So I'm to see a different doctor at the beginning of each month to have an ultrasound and see Dr. Markowich in the middle of the month to talk about it. I just don't understand why it has to be so complicated, I feel like telling her to get an ultrasound machine to examine her patients like she should, but, of course, I keep it to myself. In Turkey, they have ultrasound machines in the remotest little towns of Anatolia, how senseless it is that they make do with a single machine in this elegant, pretentious clinic in Brussels, the capital city of the EU! Well, if this is how it is, we have to go along with it. As always, we adapt to this new way of doing things easily. I jot down the dates of my next 10 or 12 appointments in my calendar and leave Dr. Markowich, without having seen the twins, to meet with her again in a month.

New Year's in Brussels

Nicole and Mark, our friends from Barcelona, had been wishing to come to Brussels to visit us for some time. We used to live very close to and see each other very often in Barcelona, but now we were separated by a long distance. We were trying to maintain our friendship even though we lived in different countries now. We had planned to meet to celebrate the New Year's together, so they came to Brussels after having celebrated Christmas with their family in Germany. As both Nicole and I were pregnant, we took advantage of the holiday to rest while our husbands did all the work. Expecting a baby doesn't just restrict your movements, it also restricts what you can eat. We were could taste neither the foie gras that Cosimo made nor the fresh oysters bought at the fish market. I sipped about half a glass of the Catalan sparkling wine Cava that Mark had brought from Barcelona, as guiltily as if I were committing a sin. I was on the pregnancy diet. I realized as I went along how many food items pregnant women were to avoid. Oh! The temptation of the forbidden fruit! I would have never missed foie gras or oysters but I craved them now that they were off the menu. I obsessed about sushi, which normally wouldn't even cross my mind...

Nicole and I spent almost the entire New Year holiday lying down and enjoying our husbands' serving and cooking for us. Food and wine were a common hobby of theirs and they liked to swap recipes and new food ideas. The New Year's menu had the traditional stuffed turkey. Mark, who was not modest about his turkey, absolutely needed a bulb baster, which we didn't have among our kitchen utensils that could possibly supply a restaurant. If you are German, and an engineer, like Mark, everything in life, even cooking, has to be perfect, everything has to be done by the book! So we had to go shopping in the morning and browse each and every store selling kitchen utensils in Brussels to find the bulb baster so the turkey could roast without drying, and the meat thermometer (no, it wouldn't do to know the oven temperature, you had to know the temperature of the turkey!), and we escaped a turkey-less New Year's! After the New Year's celebration was over and the turkey had been devoured, Mark told us about other uses for which the bulb baster might come handy. We, the two expecting mothers, listened in amazement and laughed till we cried.

It sounded almost like a joke, but it was a true story: a lesbian couple of Mark's friends who couldn't afford to go to an infertility center for artificial insemination thought the bulb baster was quite the tool for the job. Yes, exactly as you can imagine! A male homosexual friend of theirs who didn't wish to have a child and who only wanted to help his friends consented to be the sperm donor and they managed to conceive through their own method of DIY artificial insemination using the bulb baster. This story tells me that when people want to have children, the possibilities are almost endless... all over the world, even in Germany!

Longing for Barcelona

The festive season is over and life in Europe is back to its usual. Nicole and Mark have gone back to their home in Barcelona after the merry New Year's holiday we spent together. We see the doctor and do an ultrasound, which confirms that everything is alright and the twins are growing well; we are slowly approaching the happy ending. Obsessive as I am, I keep asking, "Should I be resting more? What should I be doing?" She answers calmly and assures me that there is nothing special I should be doing but what is expected of any expectant mother. "Take it easy, of course," she says, "and be watchful of anything unusual, otherwise just go on with your normal daily life."

Cosimo and I miss Barcelona and our friends there much, so we decide to take a trip, considering we might not be able to do so for a while when the twins are born. Dr. Markowich thinks it should be fine, but I still hesitate. "Really?" I keep asking, "Is it really alright if I go?" "Everything is normal," she repeats, "you may go." Is it me who is asking too many questions or is it the doctors who do not talk enough? I've seen so many doctors in my life and I still don't know the answer to this question. We time our trip so it coincides with a design exposition called "Bread & Butter" that my friend Sibel from Istanbul will also be attending. There are so many people and places I wish to see in Barcelona, but try to keep myself in check, as I made a promise to myself that I shouldn't exert myself too much on this trip, even though it's hard to keep such a promise in Barcelona. As the doctor suggested, I'm watchful of anything unusual, but I'm in the clear. My morning sickness has stopped. They say the second trimester is the most enjoyable part of pregnancy anyway, morning sickness has passed and you are not too heavy yet so you feel very energetic. In fact, I have such a surge of energy that I cannot stay put. I make an appointment to see Dr. Leila, my American doctor in Barcelona, while I'm there. I want to share the happy news with her and have her examine me. It's reassuring to see the twins on the ultrasound screen, I'm so hooked on it that I almost feel like buying an ultrasound machine to watch the twins night and day! I read in a baby magazine that I'm not alone; a Hollywood celebrity has done that – so it's not that silly an idea at all if others have done it!

Something strikes me on my way to Dr. Leila's; there are so many parents in the streets, strolling around pushing baby carriages. I didn't notice that while we lived here in Barcelona. When you are pregnant you seem to see more pregnant people or people with babies. When I see parents shopping with their babies or pushing baby carriages in the parks, I get excited and caress my belly. I cannot believe that soon, I too will be doing those things I've been longing for!

Dr. Leila is very happy to hear about the twins. I got her Pierre

Marcolini's world-famous Belgian chocolate from Brussels. She opens and holds out the black box that looks like a jewelry case with the liquor filled chocolates laid out like diamonds, and says, "This much alcohol won't hurt." We take one each and savor them "to the twins' health." Then it's time to see the babies. I miss them already even though I've seen them only ten days ago! Dr. Leila says their measurements, their movements are normal, everything is fine – words I love to hear!

The doctor's visits are like therapy for me, it reassures me to hear that they are well. I'm very happy to be in Barcelona but I can't help feeling guilty and anxious because I walk and move too much. Dr. Leila's words appease my worries a little. I've met so many doctors that I can analyze them now. I divide them into two categories; the positive ones that do you good and the negative ones that affect you worse than your ailment... just like cities which do you good or affect you badly... Barcelona is definitely one of the cities that do me good, with the sun that warms you up in mid-January, jovial people, streets filled with people in diverse, colorful clothes, cafés with crisp Manchego-and-tomato sandwiches adorning the windows, the fish market filled with the tempting smell of fresh seafood, the playful architecture and the sea. Like everything nice, our eight-day Barcelona trip must come to an end and we come back to Brussels with its wind that penetrates right to the bones. Goodbye, golden Barcelona, and hello grey Brussels...

Birth & Death

I like to read a few pages before I go to bed, it's like a sleeping pill; it mellows you out and prepares you to sleep. Reading is like daydreaming to me, it takes me to another universe. Cosimo is lying next to me, reading and caressing my protruding, widened belly. "Have you thought of names for our twins?" he asks. I have already named them in my own way, but I keep this little secret to myself. "I've been thinking," I reply. "And?" he says. I utter a few names, for which he doesn't care much. He says he likes his mother's name, to which I object, saying I wouldn't like to call my daughter with my mother-in-law's name. "Between Turkish names, Italian names, the names you like and the ones I like, we seem to be in for a hard time selecting names," he says. Touchy, under the effects of my hormones, I make an issue out of it and insist that he explains what he means. He sees that this is bound to grow out of proportion, and says he didn't mean a thing. He bids me goodnight, we gave each other a quick kiss on the lips, more of a peck, really, than a heartfelt kiss. Early in the morning tomorrow, we have an ultrasound appointment. We are going to see the twins, and that's what matters now. We will take care of names when the time comes.

I am seeing two doctors in Brussels for my prenatal care, one of them Dr. Markowich, my ob-gyn, and the other one is our ultrasound specialist, whose name I haven't managed to commit to memory yet, since I have only seen her once. I sleep very little that night, maybe because of the excitement of going to see the babies, or maybe because of our conflict about names. It's a chilly February morning. I'm standing helplessly in front of the wardrobe, thinking it's high time I go shopping for maternity clothes. I've always longed for the days where I would go shopping in the maternity department of stores, and now those days have arrived. I can't wait to go shopping. We go into the exam room.

I don't need to strip any more as it's my 19th week and sonograms can be performed externally from the fourth month onward, unless otherwise necessary. This is new information to me as I have never been past the first trimester in my previous pregnancies. I also learn that vaginal exams are more frequent during the last months as it is important to check the cervix. I lay down excitedly on the exam chair... My eyes are fixed on the dark screen. I can only make out the babies positions, the doctor will tell us the rest. He examines the image on the screen at length, without a word. Is he taking his time or is it me getting impatient? The twins keep wiggling, alive and kicking. As I tell myself to chase away bad thoughts and not to worry, the doctor says there is a problem. The baby at the bottom, the girl, has little amniotic fluid left. I blurt out questions one after another: What does this mean? What happens when there is little amniotic fluid? How little is there left? The doctor just keeps examining attentively, without really answering me. He says Dr. Markowich needs to see me. Luckily, Dr. Markowich is in the hospital for a delivery, so they send me to the Edith Cavell straight away.

We are waiting for the doctor to come out of the delivery room. They take me into a room and ask me to remove all my clothes, put on a hospital gown and wait lying down – this must be serious. The minutes seem to linger on. I'm seized by cold fear all over, I'm freezing, and finally I burst into tears. Cosimo tries to calm me down to no avail, he too is very upset and anxious. Dr. Markowich shows up at last, obviously aware of my condition, she's at a loss, she doesn't seem to know what to say... When I ask whether I will lose the babies, she says, "It's serious. But it's too early to tell, yet. Let's do a test first and then we can evaluate the case according to the results."

They take me on the gurney to another room for ob-gyn interventions. Dr. Markowich reads the instructions on the box of the test kit carefully as if she were doing it for the first time, saying, "It's a new test, we used to have other methods." There's a piece of paper in the kit, resembling litmus paper that's supposed to change color when it comes into contact with amniotic fluid. They will check whether there is any loss of amniotic fluid and whether the cervix has started dilating. I keep saying prayers in my mind, unable to believe what's happening.

As she's examining the paper, Dr. Markowich tries to explain the basics of the situation: "The amniotic membranes normally rupture just before labor and the amniotic fluid* is released. This is what they call it 'when your water breaks' and it's a sign that the baby is coming. It can vary from woman to woman, in some cases the membranes do not rupture until the last moment. It's only one of the many signs of labor. Unfortunately, there is a tiny perforation in the amniotic sac of the twin at the bottom, from where the amniotic fluid has leaked out and is almost depleted. The baby needs that fluid to grow. Furthermore, since it's a sign of labor, it signals the cervix to start dilating, and once the cervix

----

* Amniotic fluid is the liquid that helps protect the baby from external influences. The embryo swallows this sweetish fluid and excretes it back through the kidneys, thus both consuming and producing it at the same time. The baby does its first exercises to develop swallowing skills and muscle control in this fluid, starting as early as in the first months. The amount of fluid, which is around 100 ml in the third month, goes up to 1.5 liters towards the end of the pregnancy and drops to about 800 ml a short while before labor due to the cramped space.

is dilated you and the babies will be vulnerable to infection. A woman cannot and should not carry on with pregnancy for long under such conditions. It's very hazardous for her health."

It's like a dark joke, almost surreal. So, is that it? Is this how the life of the twins, who have been growing up nice and healthily, will end? I try not to think about it, I don't want to think about it, but I can't help the voice in my mind, ceaselessly accusing me of having done something wrong and I cannot stop crying...

I talked to Dr. Markowich on the phone only a few days ago. How stupid I am! I thought I had a urinary tract infection; it didn't occur to me that the fluid that kept dripping when I went to the toilet was amniotic fluid. I called my doctor and told her that I wanted to come in for an exam immediately as I had a discharge and suspected urinary tract infection, so we arranged a visit on the date of my ultrasound appointment in three days, but she asked me to go to the laboratory first for a test and told me she would call me when she had the results. I did as I was told and waited for her call. The next day her assistant called me to say the test results showed no sign of infection, and I dismissed my worries as one of the typical cases of paranoia I tend to experience when I'm pregnant, telling myself, 'Come on, Nur. Calm down! All is well. This must be one of those things women go through when they are expecting.' I remembered reading in What to Expect When You Are Expecting, the pregnant women's bible, that the growing uterus puts pressure on the bladder, making you feel constantly as if you have to go.

What I thought was urine was in fact the amniotic fluid,

leaking from the perforated sac of my baby girl nestled in the lower part of my womb, and she cannot be expected to make it until the end of the pregnancy with the little fluid left. The babies are so small there is nothing to do, we are medically unable to make them survive. A 20-week old baby's lungs are not adequately developed to allow it to breathe when it's born. The survival limit is normally 28 weeks, from which point onwards a baby can survive in an incubator. Younger babies born prematurely can sometimes be kept alive. There was a 24-week old baby born in Brussels that was kept in an incubator and made it, but it's very rare and very risky.

I cannot accept the thought of losing the twins. No! They cannot just slip through my fingers, there must be something we can do. My son, in the upper part of my womb, is fine, growing healthily, but he has to go, too! I cannot begin to understand how come they cannot save him, are we going to end his life, just like that! Why, but why? I wonder how they cannot do anything about it with so many modern medical technologies. But they say it's too great of a risk to allow for a woman go through with her pregnancy in a case like this, as it jeopardizes the life of the mother trying to save the healthy baby.

A friend of mine had conceived twin babies through in vitro fertilization. All was going well when they found out one of the babies had a genetic problem hindering its healthy growth and it was terminated. Since she was three-months pregnant, her body just made away with one baby while the other baby remained. Then she went on with her pregnancy without any other problems and gave birth to a healthy baby. The reason why they cannot solve my problem is that I'm in the fifth month of my pregnancy: too early to deliver, too late to leave one of the twins behind and go on!

My Hospital Diary

I'm admitted to the hospital for an uncertain period of time; it can be anything from two weeks to two months, or even until delivery... I don't have the slightest objection to being in a hospital as long as my babies are fine. My doctor will discuss the issue with the other obstetricians in the hospital and they will decide the best way to proceed for my babies and me. The only thing to do at the moment is to wait (for at least a week) and see. As the baby girl's sac is perforated I am not to move at all and have to stay in bed all the time. We will see if the level of amniotic liquid rises... There have been cases where the amniotic fluid was seen to increase in women who were six or seven months pregnant and had similar problems, and their babies grew up to be born healthy. What wouldn't I give to be one of those success stories!

Cosimo and I inform our families without getting into much detail. There is no point in upsetting them at this point, the two of us are upset anyway. My mother asks me whether I would like her to come at once, to which I can hardly say no. She jumps on the plane and comes straight away. Dearest mother! She's always there when I need her. My darling husband Cosimo is there too, waiting on me hand and foot. He understands how I feel lying in bed in a hospital room and does everything he can to cheer me up. He keeps bringing me things like an ant stocking its nest, he brings my books, my laptop, my magazines, my moisturizers, basically everything I need from home, so the drawers and cabinets in my hospital room are crammed.

I don't really have time to read all those books and magazines anyway. It may sound like a joke, but when you are in the hospital you don't have much time left to get bored; your day is filled with exams, monitoring, and treatment activities. My mother is always with me during the day, then Cosimo comes in after work and they go back home together in the evening since there is no bed for a visitor in the room. There is only a (slightly) reclining chair but I don't think it's meant to serve as a bed. I don't need anyone to stay with me at night anyway, as there are at least four nurses on call in the obstetrics ward, who appear by your bedside the moment you need them. Yes, a hospital is a hospital and there is a limit up to which it can be comfortable. But the Edith Cavell is almost a boutique hotel; you cannot be uncomfortable in there. They do everything to keep me at ease.

My busy daily hospital routine is about the same every day. First, I make an early start with breakfast served at seven o'clock, before it's even daylight. Frankly, it's not bad at all to wake up to a nice and hot cup of tea that comes in a thermos. After breakfast, the nurses give me a sponge bath in bed, as I'm not allowed to get up, let alone take a shower. I cannot grasp how they do it but they change the bed sheet with unbelievable efficiency while I'm lying on it! The bed linen smells of fresh Marseille soap. I have a very particular sense of smell and the peculiar habit of sniffing everything, much like our dog Çakır does. Fortunately for me, the hospital is extremely fastidious about cleanliness and odors, exactly what I need! When the morning cleaning is completed, the nurses come to take my temperature and blood pressure. Then another nurse comes pulling a non-stress test (NST) device on a wheel table. She rubs a cold gel on my abdomen and puts two belts around my belly, one for each of the twins. She tries to locate the babies' heartbeats, moving the devices on the belts on my belly, until finally she hears the noise resembling that of a horse's gallop and fixes the device on that spot. The monitors are connected to the device on the wheeled table, which prints a continuous graph of the babies' movements and heartbeats on a long paper ribbon that keeps coming out of the machine and sprawling on the ground. I have to stay pretty motionless for at least 20 minutes, otherwise the monitors on my belly might move and we might have to start all over again.

I'm now pretty used to lying still anyway, I only sit up a little bit when I'm eating and I lie on my side when I sleep, as I cannot possibly sleep on my back. It's not easy to turn on my side either, I try not to lift my body and move too much. After the procedure the nurses take the graphics to my doctor. Then the door opens again and a nurse takes a blood sample to test for infection. Lunch is served just before noon. As the breakfast consisting of two slices of bread, a small packet of butter and some jelly is bland, and not very satisfying, I'm ready for an early lunch, which, fortunately, is quite rich. I find the meal times to be the most exciting time of the hospital day. In the afternoon, I have another NST session, and, again, the results are taken to the doctor. My temperature and blood pressure are taken, and then it's tea time. It's dull to have your last meal of the day at such an early hour. The menu consists of bland dishes, probably so that patients having to lie down all the time can digest their meal easily. Tea is over at an early hour.

The nights are long, I have time, but somehow I cannot concentrate either on reading or on writing. My mind is permanently busy with the twins. The nurses advise me to sleep and rest but on the other hand they won't give me a minute's break, knocking on my door continually day and night and expecting me to answer. Not that they would heed if I told them not to come in! They knock just as a matter of habit. The flux of people coming in and out of the room to perform tests or treatments, to take out the garbage, or just by mistake never seems to stop. In addition, they are renovating part of the hospital. My room has already been done but there is always something missing or not functioning properly so the repairmen just cannot stay away. Not to mention the drilling and hammering noises from the neighboring rooms!

It's impossible to sleep with this racket, but I really like daytime naps anyway, I like to sleep after midnight. It seems to me it's a waste of time to sleep in during the day, when it's light outside and there's so much to do. But I wouldn't mind being able to sleep the days away now that I'm in the hospital, maybe it would help me and stop me from worrying. Fortunately, I often have friends coming to visit me, they don't leave me for a minute. It's been only six months since we moved to Brussels but we've already met such lovely people both from Cosimo's workplace and through our friends from Istanbul that it's almost as if we were surrounded by old friends. Emotional as I am, I shed tears talking to each and every one of my visitors, which helps me vent the negative feelings in a way. Friends who live far keep calling on the phone and trying to cheer me up.

My childhood friend Umut happens to be in Paris on a business trip and we often talk on the phone. Even though Brussels is very close to Paris, I cannot expect her to come when she's so busy, but this is what friends are like, they don't care about time or distance. I've just put my book down and turned my night light off that there's a knock on the door. I'm a little annoyed thinking it's the nurses again when a face shows up at the door. I cannot make it out at first, although it looks very familiar. Dear Umut, she's standing there with a smile from ear to ear and her blue eyes glittering sagely even in the night. It's the best surprise ever! We locked in a giant embrace. "I cannot believe it!" I say, to which she replies, "Believe it, it's me, here I am. I just had to see and talk to you. You won't be alone tonight." I ask how much time we have together, as there is so much to catch up on. "I'll be with you till morning," she says. We talk the night away, until we're out of breath. We don't talk much about the twins, she senses what I need and takes me away to another world from the hospital. She stays with me for seven hours, during which we laugh a lot.

When they knock on the door to bring in my breakfast, Umut just jumps up from the reclining chair where she's had a few hours' nap, dynamic and energetic as ever, goes to the mirror to tidy herself up, puts on her red lipstick and fixes her blond curls. She is ready for the day, as if she hasn't been up all night! "I'm going to the train station, now," she says. "You must miss being outside, is there anything you'd like for me to do?" I say, "Yes, I've always wanted to take you to the Pain Quotidien. I want you go and have a nice breakfast there for both of us." "Gladly," she replies and we give each other a long hug, inhaling each other's scent. She gives me a big kiss on the cheek before she leaves me, saying, "Don't worry, my dear, it's all going to be fine soon." I drift into the mellow memories of happy old days until the first nurse of the morning comes in and pricks me with a needle to collect a blood sample, reminding me I'm still in a hospital.

There is heavy traffic today right from the very early morning.
Our landlord Jean Pierre, who is an early bird like me, calls around
eight o'clock. "Just heard the news... How are you, sister?" (We
call each other sister and brother.) I dissolve in tears as soon as I
hear his voice, which I can hear cracking on the other end of the
line. "Don't," he says. "You'll make me cry, too." Jean Pierre is one
of the most sentimental people I've ever known. His real name
is Nurettin, he is from Tunisian origin but he went to Paris to
study when he was young and later settled in Brussels. He told
me he was fiftyish when we first met but I believe he must be
around sixty years old. He's a looker, with a fit body and a botoxed
face. He's very energetic, always on the move; he could run rings
around young people. He lives alone most of time and sometimes
with a girlfriend who constantly keeps changing. He always says
he hasn't had children because he has never met the right woman,
tells me to find him a Turkish girl like me to marry and then
complains, "No, no, marriage isn't for me, I'm happy as I am."

He asks me if he can come and visit me in the hospital and
whether I need anything. In an hour, he turns up with our cleaning
lady, a Romanian girl called Melanie, who was at Jean Pierre's that
morning and wanted to come with him when she heard he was
coming to see me. I very happy to see them. Melanie used to bring
me cookies and pies of all kinds every time she came to work
in the house so the twins would grow stronger. And this time,
Jean Pierre has brought me a huge box of assorted sushi from his
favorite Japanese restaurant. He couldn't be expected to know that
expectant mothers are not allowed to consume raw fish and I don't
want to tell him and hurt his feelings, so I tell a white lie and say
"I'll have them for lunch."

I've been in the hospital for a week. They have me lie at an angle of probably 30 degrees, if not 45, with my head down, which causes me to feel as if all my blood goes to my brain. It's very unpleasant but I'm ready to do anything. It's supposed to stop the loss of amniotic fluid and maybe allow it to increase. I have to increase my fluid intake and I'm not allowed to stand or even sit. I eat my meals lying upside down and I use a bedpan to relieve myself. However unpleasant it is to have someone I don't even know to wash down my private parts, there is nothing I can do to help it. Now I understand so well the feelings of patients confined to bed for a lifetime! You've got to thank God every single day for what you have, that's all there is to life!

I do an ultrasound at the end of the first week. I've been drinking nonstop for a whole week now, water, tea, herbal teas, coffee, milk, and fruit juices, whatever comes my way. Women normally hate it when they drink too much and their belly bulges, but when it's for the baby nothing else matters; we agree to drink until we burst and to swell like a balloon. We roam the hospital corridors with a gurney; it's not the nurses that push it, there are special gurney drivers to do this job, it requires quite a skill level! The doctor who conducts the sonogram tells me only that the babies are well and writes a note containing the rest of the information to my doctor, which she puts in an envelope and places on the gurney.

The gurney driver comes to drive me back to my room through the long corridors. I examine the sonogram pictures trying to find out if there is any increase in my baby girl's fluid level. There is a glimmer of hope in me, I keep thinking they will live. I study the pictures fixedly until the nurses come and take the file from me to hand it to my doctor, they say something like, "Your doctor will soon be here to see you." in French. It's a good thing I took that course, I've found an opportunity to practice my French in here, although I'd have preferred to practice in a café rather than a hospital. The daily hospital routine goes on. Usually my doctor visits me in the room in the morning to evaluate the situation, then goes on to visit her other patients in the maternity ward. She seems to be spending more time with me, which may be because I'm in such a delicate condition. Today is an important day as it will be decided whether or not I can go on with my pregnancy, depending on the evaluation of sonogram results.

My eyes are fixed on the door as I am waiting for Dr. Markowich, counting the minutes. Today she comes in during the afternoon. I can sense she's having difficulty broaching the subject. She seems to be self-conscious and maybe feels a little guilty since didn't give me an appointment when I called her, concerned with a possible urinary tract infection. She tells me there is no change in the amniotic fluid level and, unfortunately, we don't seem to have any other options but to terminate the pregnancy. She adds, turning her eyes away, "Two of my fellow physicians and I agree on that... of course, you're welcome to get another doctor's opinion." Even the doctor seems to have lost her professional composure talking to me. You can tell she's upset. I'm so helpless, so desperate at this moment that I'm ready to try anything to save the twins. I decide to call Dr. De Catte, who takes care of critical pregnancy cases in the AZ-VUB hospital, and who I think is more experienced in such cases. I call and tell her everything and ask her opinion. Naturally, she says she will have to see me, so I leave the Edith Cavell with my treatment file, my twins in my belly and my hopes of saving them.

The Ambulance & Despair...

It always makes my hair stand on end to hear an ambulance passing by. I visualize the patient lying on the gurney in the ambulance, injured or fighting for his life. Now I am that patient. There is no need to sound the siren as this is not an emergency; I'm only being transported to another hospital. Still, the driver decides to sound it when he sees the traffic in the tunnel. So the siren is not sounded only for patients fighting for their lives, I thank God. But then I might prefer to be injured than to have to suffer this. Yes, definitely, I would. I could bear my own pain more easily than having to say farewell to the two babies in my womb. For a moment, I think of the people who lose their loved ones slowly to some disease, who have to watch them slip through their fingers. The helplessness must be harder to endure than the pain! And I feel so helpless, so hopeless now while I'm being driven to another hospital. My hands are tied, there is nothing I can do, and it kills me. I revolt against this law of the nature – if it is the law of the nature – which I cannot begin to understand! But I can understand now why people either devote themselves to religion or fall out of it when they are faced with such tragedies.

❦

It feels like I'm back to the beginning. I'm in AZ-VUB (Academische Ziekenhuis Vrije Universiteit Brussels) Hospital and Doctor De Catte isn't saying anything different from the doctors in Et Cavell Hospital. My waters having broken means that the membranes are ruptured and the cervix is ready for birth and that I'm vulnerable to infection if birth is delayed, which is, so I'm told, very dangerous. In some cases where the expectant mother is of an older age, and the odds of her conceiving again are low, it is possible to remove the twin with the ruptured amniotic sack from the womb and let the mother go on with the pregnancy with the unaffected baby. But the remaining gestation period is a long, difficult, and risky time, and the expectant mother has to spend the rest of her pregnancy in the hospital. The eight days that I've had to spend in the hospital seemed so long that I feel those who stay for months should be given a medal!

The doctor has explained the situation and told us that birth is our best option in this situation. 'Birth' is only a technical term. The twins are only 20 weeks old and won't survive. In other words, their birth will also be their death. Their organs and especially their lungs not having developed yet, they won't be able to breathe. It's so painful to even pronounce the word death! Or I might try the other option, which is to say goodbye to my baby girl with the ruptured sack and embark on a long and risky process. As I am 36, my doctor thinks I stand a good chance of conceiving again. I have to make a quick decision and my doctor is clearly encouraging me to go for the abortion of both twins. Thinking reasonably, it does make sense, yet the mere thought is breaking my heart. I cannot bear to think that they are alive in my belly and that their life will be over once they are born. What have I done wrong? I keep having flashbacks, trying to visualize what I have done or been through during the last days and blaming myself.

Cosimo and I are alone in the hospital room and talk privately. My dearest husband holds my hand softly and gives me a kiss on the lips and tells me I am the most important being on earth to him. "We cannot risk your life for the baby," he says. "The decision, of course, is yours to make, but we mustn't act emotionally." Even if I decide to keep the unaffected twin I must acknowledge that I am taking a risk and accept the hardship that will follow. The baby might catch an infection, develop complications and be unhealthy. Inducing 'birth' seems to be the right thing to do.

I still remember the hours, even the minutes before the birth so vividly... I felt like a mother who had acquiesced to euthanasia for her children. Although I had never seen them, never lived with them, they had been a part of me for five months and I had bonded with them. If it hurt that much to end five months of such a connection I couldn't even start to imagine how painful the loss of a child would be to a mother who had nursed, raised and reared it! Burying her children must be the utmost torment in life for a mother.

I'm never alone in my room at the hospital, people keep coming and going with explanations, statements, papers to be read and signed... numerous tasteless formalities. Do I have to deal with all this right at this moment? Fortunately, I meet the psychologist from the ob-gyn department. (I'm impressed with the hospital; you can tell they take this to heart.) He first asks how I am. How could I be? He tells me I can see him if I need assistance. I cannot predict how I will feel or whether I'll need anything once all this is over. The psychologist embarks on whether I would like to take the babies or leave them with the hospital after the birth. AZ-VUB is a hospital that takes care of patients of a variety of religious affiliations. Since they know I am Muslim they think I might wish to hold a funeral, which, honestly, has never even crossed my mind. It would be meaningless for me to have gravestones erected for them as they were never born. And it would hurt me more to bury them if I saw them. Cosimo asks the question I cannot bring myself to ask: "What do you do with them if we don't take them?"

"The hospital has a..." I don't want to hear! The psychologist senses my discomfort, apologetically, he says he needs to go through with this procedure and have the answers on record before the birth, and goes on with his questions: "Would you like to see the twins when they are born? Seeing the babies may help the mother to have closure. This is what we recommend you do, but it is up to you to decide." The psychologist insists that I see them, suggesting it would actually help me. Maybe it does work for some but it just isn't for me, I refuse. "You may not want to see them now but you might change your mind later," he says. "We take pictures of the babies when they are born and we archive them, so you'll still have the chance to see them even years after the birth."

I wouldn't know about other mothers but personally, I would only find it upsetting to see their tiny, lifeless bodies, I knew that. I still feel the same and I don't wish to see them, their pictures may remain in the archives as their image will remain in my memory and their love in my heart...

The birth is to be induced via a simple vaginal suppository. They must have figured the birth would come through the next morning if they applied the suppository around six o'clock in the evening. I ask when the contractions will start. My doctor tells me that it might take as long as 36 hours. "You relax now," he suggests. "You try to get some sleep. I'll see you in the morning." And he leaves the room with flatfooted doctor's steps before I can even start to ask "What if, while you're away..." I turn to the nurses with my question: "What if my contractions start during the night? Will you call the doctor for the birth?" One of the nurses, seeing the alarm in my face, gives me a nod that I find far from being reassuring. The other one says she will call the doctor on call so I can talk to her.

A lovely, young lady comes in... She is so young I almost can't believe she has studied medicine and specialized in gynecology. "I've been told you are Turkish," she says, in Turkish! She has a slight accent but she does look Turkish, so I ask whether she is. "No, I am Belgian, my husband is Turkish, I learned Turkish from him," she answers. Her husband is from Agri. I congratulate her, saying "My husband is Italian and we have been married for six and a half years. He can only construct simple sentences in Turkish. Either I have failed in teaching him or he is not really interested in learning." As we start to talk about Turkey and Turkish people I forget about the things I meant to ask the doctor, which I am reminded by the onset of slight contractions. I'm a woman with such a high threshold of pain that I might almost give birth without anyone noticing. The contractions start getting stronger and more frequent. I think the expected moment is there... At 9.30 I am admitted to the delivery room.

My doctor can't make it to the delivery. I knew it anyway. For some reason I feel like I have given birth before. I knew when I was induced that the contractions would start very soon and I'd be in labor straight away and I was annoyed that the doctor didn't wait up to see it through. I am tired of explaining myself to different doctors each time, I wish a familiar doctor would come to assist the delivery. There are two gynecologists on call, one is the young doctor I've met. She is only 26. She is not a GP or an intern, she is actually an ob-gyn specialist. The other one I have never met. Questions such as "Can this be the young doctor's first delivery?" and "Am I going to be her first experience?" add to my fear of birth. But when she looks at me and says "Don't worry, calm down," in her nice, soft voice and her Turkish with an eastern accent, I feel I can trust her. I find myself oddly calm and peaceful.

The anxiety I've felt until then recedes to a strange peace and happiness, a false sense of contentment pervades my mind, I am excited as if I were to have my babies soon. My mind and body are numb like I have been drinking. It must be the effect of the epidural.* I know they are now alive in my womb and that they will die as soon as they are out but I feel oddly wonderful, I experience a spurious joy of motherhood, maybe it is the experience of that indescribable moment of fulfillment where my urge to be a mother is satisfied, where a missing part of me becomes whole...

Then the babies leave my womb one after the other, their tiny bodies are wrapped in white sheets and taken to the room next

---

* To relieve pain during labor, a method called epidural anesthesia is used, where a drug is injected to your lower back, leaving you numbed from the waist down, as if you were paralyzed. But your pelvic muscles that will do the work during labor remain active. You remain conscious and can see and feel everything that goes on during delivery, yet feel no pain; which leaves you with nice memories of the moment of birth. We are a lucky generation. Our mothers went through so much pain when they gave birth to us, so much has changed since then. They had told us about the difficulties and the pain of child birth, now everything seems to have become easier but it's actually harder to have a baby.

door by the nurses. Right then the false sense of happiness vanishes and a vast emptiness remains in my belly, and my heart. They are now gone. My husband is near me, he says, although he didn't want to see them, he hasn't been able to look away while they were being taken to the exam room and he has seen them, though not very closely. I have felt their warmth, their bodies slide away from mine; that bodily perception was much more satisfactory than just seeing them. The delivery is easily and quickly through. The young gynecologist and the two nurses congratulate me for giving birth to the twins with just two pushes, which I know is a kind of consolation; they are trying to comfort me as they can anticipate what I'll be going through after the delivery.

An Empty House...

I could never forget the moment I came home from the hospital. I'd probably never felt sadder. When I'd left home two weeks ago to go to my monthly prenatal appointment I didn't even suspect that I'd be coming back empty handed and broken. I'd never had any experience that affected me like that in my 36 years of life. Sorrow teaches you many things. I didn't know what it meant to hit the bottom. Now I was so low that I could really understand the meaning of being depressed. Our vast living room of 40 square meters was oppressing me, the big white couch I used to love to sink in didn't feel comfortable, I collapsed in it like a heavy, lifeless mass, feeling exhausted. I was looking around the room from where I sat, doing nothing. Everything seemed so vain, devoid of meaning, it felt as though nothing would ever be the same again. I had built my future plans on the twins. I, my life, my home, were now nothing but a huge vacuum. What was I supposed to do now? Where was I supposed to find the strength to start all over again?

At that depressed period of my life, I found solace in novels, in similar life stories to mine, and in stories I heard from people around me. One day, when I was zapping through the TV channels, I came across the story of a village woman living in East Anatolia on a Turkish channel, who had used a micro-credit to set up her own business in a small town. She made and sold sieves and seemed to be quite happy with herself, telling she struggled with poverty before she had started this business but she was now able to put bread on the table for her children at least. She had lost nine babies and then had four children. You had to bow to her vital power and look up to her. Being pregnant nine times, burying the babies you'd been carrying in your womb as soon as they were born, and trying again, and again, without faltering, without wavering with the doubt that you might lose them again, without losing hope... what kind of strength did it take? I would like to meet that woman, to listen to what she'd been through, to learn about her feelings. We had lost two babies and were shattered, but her... I couldn't even bring myself to say it, my heart went out to her. There was so much sorrow, so much pain and misery everywhere, I was witnessing the suffering of people in other countries and other homes...

Avoiding Happiness

I find it easy to express, to write about my happy feelings, whereas I've always been bad at expressing my sadness. I've never thought why until now, until I've been this badly shaken by this losing the twins. Maybe I wish to dismiss the things that make me unhappy, erase them from memory or cover them up... Maybe I don't want to bother others with my sorrow...

I feel miserable, so miserable, I've never been more so in my life. I used to think I was a happy person, consider myself lucky to have been born far away from all the misery, all the wars that plague the earth, even though I sometimes shadowed my happiness with superfluous anxieties. I know I'll get over this and get back to my old, happy mood but I cannot help worrying. My husband has also been traumatized, he too is very sad... It's hard to tell which one of us is sadder, but we are both obviously inconsolable. He sulks all the time, he lets little things get to him. He sometimes lets phrases like "How unlucky I am!" or "What an unlucky couple we are!" slip after which he apologizes and comes snuggling up to me like a cat asking for attention.

My dear friends Sibel and Yılmaz come from Turkey to give us support. My mother is still staying with us... They don't leave our sides for a minute. We are surrounded by people who care about us. When they tell me I'm recovering, I feel better, I feel my joie de vivre revive in me. It looks like Cosimo's going to take some more time to heal. Isn't love powerful: when I see him like that I forget my own misery and feel sorry for him, I can't stand seeing him like that. I have to do something for him.

Winter is a long, cold, depressing season in Brussels, the sky is slate grey. But we need light, sun, and melatonin. It's early March and it's raining even in Morocco, so we can't find ourselves a warm holiday destination in the Mediterranean. To find a sunny beach in mid-winter, you have to travel almost down to the equator. I go at once to the nearest travel agency for information. The Belgians' most popular holiday destination during winter is Senegal, a West African country that you can reach directly from Brussels with a five and a half hour flight. With an average temperature of 27 degrees Celsius throughout the year, it's a great place to visit no matter the season. It has a coastline on the Atlantic Ocean. The sea is not all that spectacular but the beach is vast. The west of the county is covered with nothing but rolling sandy plains. It's mid-winter, being on a sandy beach and watching the sea would be enough, in fact I might make do with just putting my toes in the sea! Lying on loungers, basking in the sun, our minds free from care and sorrow; that's our fantasy holiday...

And Senegal

So we decide to do like Belgians do and go to Senegal for a break. Senegal is a former French colony. If you go to a holiday village and spend your entire holiday in there, you will come back without the slightest notion about the country and Africa. It's the same as any holiday village you might find in Antalya. You will eat, drink, bask in the sun, make small talk with the European guests – most of whom are French and Belgian – during the open buffet, and endure the European music performed by a pianist singer throughout dinner... I've never enjoyed too much comfort and, free spirited as I am, never been able to come to terms with the discipline of the holiday villages. Cosimo and I spend two days lying in lounge chairs at the beach, sipping exotic cocktails, at the end of which we decide we've had enough of it and make friends with a local man.

We have to explore Senegal. We travel around the country with two cameras and a guide, in a vehicle they call a jeep but which I could only describe as a tin box with wheels, leaving no town or village unseen. We even visit our Senegalese friend's humble home, consisting of a single room serving both as living room and bed room, and kitchen, furnished with a simple couch. They have placed the most important object of the house, the TV set, at the nicest corner of the room, on their best furniture. Roaming in the streets in the village, in all the houses of which I can have a glimpse through the open doors, I see the same thing: a television placed on a high shelf on the wall and kids and youths watching it... The woman's duty is the same as it is all over the world: to feed the family.

Most women are waiting in line for water, with pails or cans on their shoulders, some are removing the stones from their rice in their courtyards or stirring old pots all black at the bottom on open fires. As we converse, they tell us that tourists love their country and come back time and time again, whereas the local youths want to escape from it. They ask us if we have come for the sea. I tell them I lost my twin babies and took this trip as I thought a change might do me good. They say, "It's lucky you survived; it's common here that the pregnant women die with their babies." It reminds me of an article I've read, the figures are in fact disheartening. A pregnant woman is 180 times more likely to die in Africa than in Western Europe. Isn't the earth a strange place? People who don't have the means and the proper physical conditions to have children have rows of them while people who do cannot have children.

I have my period for the first time after delivery. How unlucky it coincides with our holiday, and comes on a particularly inconvenient time. We are on a boat trip organized by the holiday village, where we are going to visit a number of small islands. It's too late when I realize the white sarong I'm wearing on my bathing suit is stained with blood! I'm sure everybody in our group of fifteen knows I have my period, I bet some even think I should be so reckless to let this happen. But I've forgotten about this female routine during my five month pregnancy and never thought it would come back in as short as a month after delivery. If the sharks in the Atlantic Ocean can smell blood we are in trouble! Honestly, it's the first time something like this is happening to me, a bloodbath in the literal sense of the word. I manage by staying in the sea all the time. What I regret most is that I cannot have a nice soak in the tub in our romantic bungalow and that, because of my untimely period, we cannot take advantage of this holiday to rekindle our romantic life, which has been pretty dull for the last six months anyway.

Bitten by the Africa Bug!

The people of Senegal took me back to my childhood with their lifestyle, attitudes and clothing. People wearing bright colored clothes, walking with confidence when they were treading the rough dirt roads in their dusty shoes looked like they were defying poverty. They were poor, yes, but they had smiles on their faces. Just like the people in the Gypsy quarter in Tekirdağ during my childhood... They lived life outside, on the streets rather than inside their homes, the women strolled the streets gaily, all dressed up. African women were tall and attractive, and absolutely beautiful in their modernized traditional clothes, a beauty they didn't try to hide. Young mothers, flamboyantly dressed up in spite of their having a young baby, carried their babies strapped up on their back, so the babies grew up fastened to their mother. They were able to do their daily jobs while the baby was strapped on their chest or back. When the baby was hungry, they placed it on the pouch that they formed out of a piece of cloth on their belly like a kangaroos pouch and were able to breastfeed and walk at the same time. The babies seemed to be happy about this arrangement as I saw not even one crying baby. When the baby started to walk, he could play outside with his friends and grow freely. The Senegalese who never failed to smile in spite of their poverty amazed me with their lifestyle which should set an example to all Muslim countries. Senegal is a secular country, where the majority of the population is Muslim although there are also Christians. They all live in peace together. At least for today, and I hope, forever...

What the Europeans, especially the French and the Belgians, call the Africa bug is not the malaria-carrying mosquito as you may have thought, but the longing for Africa and the wish to go back when you have left it. Yes, I was bitten by the Africa bug.* I was already planning my next trip to Africa! Besides, it was the perfect place to practice my French, as people loved to talk in here whereas people in Brussels are not very talkative.

* *In reality, our trip to Senegal was not a calm and relaxing holiday. My husband was sad, and seemed to only enjoy the moments where he was riding a jet-ski or at the spa. I, on the other hand, wasn't*

happy with the way I looked in a bathing suit with my breasts still swollen with milk, my fat thighs and sagging belly, and felt even more bloated under the sun. The reason for my bloating became apparent soon, with the unexpected arrival of my period. With the addition of mosquito bites, my whole body swelled up like a balloon. On our way back to Brussels, my residence permit (the kind given to people who arrived recently to Belgium) was not accepted and I was detained from flying into Brussels. I was told that, as I was going to fly from Africa to Europe, I could only fly to Spain because I still had a valid residence permit, and could go to Brussels from there. Now, I wouldn't have had to deal with any of this had the snail-slow Italian embassy issued my Italian passport. So I had to fly to the Canary Islands, then to Madrid, and then to Brussels, extending a normally five-hour journey to almost 24 hours. Would I still like to go back to Senegal? Why not? I just can't help it, I'm an incurable Pollyanna and a chronic adventure-loving traveler.

Travel Therapy

We were back home after our thrilling return trip from Senegal. It was nice to be home. But spring was here and we couldn't stay put. One trip triggered another and we yielded ourselves to our desire to travel. Exploring new places seemed to alleviate our grief, or maybe we were unconsciously fleeing our home, our usual environment, fleeing the reality. Who knows? Brussels' geographical location allowed us to travel easily, which we put to good use. The high speed train trip to Paris took 1 hour and 20 minutes, to London, about 2 hours. Driving to Luxembourg took an hour and a half, and to Germany, around 2 hours, and it took about three hours to go Amsterdam as there was no high speed rail yet. What I preferred was to have a lunch break in Antwerp, the city of design, then to drive to Rotterdam, a city with impressive architecture, and one of my favorite. We planned to spend a night in Hotel New York and from there to drive to Amsterdam.

I felt a little lighter, a little more relieved after each trip we took. It also motivated me to make changes in my life, which was a good sign*. But I was still having frequent mood swings and kept asking myself the same questions over and over again: Why me? Why did all the unfortunate odds always happen to me? Was I not going to make it, was I never to have a baby? These pessimistic questions were hard to answer. The other expecting mothers I'd met while I was expecting were now raising their babies. I was so sensitive about that that I couldn't find the strength to go see my friends' new born babies even though I really wanted to. When my Norwegian classmate's baby was born, I paid them a visit, and naturally we talked of nothing but the baby, which shook me deeply. I wasn't ready for any further visits. My wound was still fresh, for quite a while to go seeing a newborn baby was going to remind me of my twins. I had to give myself some more time. I was rushing aging, as I always did.

---

* I am a travel-holic, but my favorite thing about traveling is coming back home. I always miss my life, my home, my routine when I'm away traveling and dream about the things I'll take up when I'm back, because travelling inspires my artistic spirit, and allows me to look back at my life from a distance, so I can examine the things that are not right and need changing.

The Life Coach

For a long time, I couldn't keep myself from crying. I used to wake up in the morning deprived from any sense of purpose. I had periods where I didn't set my foot outside and spend the entire day in my pajamas. For some time, I didn't feel like doing anything. How incredible it was that a social butterfly like me was turned into an unsociable person who didn't want to see or talk to anyone! When I was only a child, my mother used to say, "My daughter could make friends with the birds in the sky!" I had the gift of connecting to people easily. I was sure this isolation tendency would soon pass, which it did. One morning, I got up feeling better. I took a shower. I gave myself a once-over in the mirror; it looked as if I was starting to lose the extra pounds. I tried on some of the trousers I used to wear before pregnancy, and I could almost do the buttons. I dressed up and put my make-up on. I had a feeling that a nice day awaited me, even though it was grey outside. It was time to go back to normal, to look ahead and think about my life and my goals.

When we had first moved to Brussels, I had read all the expat magazines and newspapers, trying to adapt to a new city and a new life and looking for pursuits that could help me make connections. I was interested in language courses, or design courses that could help me in my profession. When I studied architecture, we used to include garden landscapes in our projects, it could be an idea to take a landscape design course, as Belgium was all about horticulture and garden design. But the courses required a high proficiency of French language. So I decided to improve my French. While I was browsing through the pages, an ad caught my eye: It was the ad of a career center helping professionals who had come to Belgium for various reasons and who didn't have a job. I attended a few publicity meetings but I couldn't pursue it any further when I got pregnant with the twins.

I thought it might be a good idea to apply to that center to find out about the business opportunities in Brussels. I called straight away and made an appointment with the life coach recommended by the secretary who answered the phone. While I sat in the library of the center, browsing the books, I overheard the conversation of two girls working there, one British and one Polish. The Polish girl was three months pregnant and was already thinking about where she was going to go for the delivery, how they had to move to a larger house before the baby came and how she wanted to decorate the nursery. I was mad at myself for not being able to help envying her. She was confident that she was going to have a baby and very comfortable with her plans about the future. She was so relaxed! How different our cares and concerns were! She worried about the color scheme to use in the nursery when I was constantly troubled with the fear of loss during my pregnancies. It seemed impossible for me to shake off these thoughts and go back to being who I used to be. I knew the solution was in me, somewhere inside me. All I needed was motivation. Losses and failures had pushed me into a state of apathy.

The life coach of the career center, Paul, an American of Japanese origin, helped me a lot. The first life coach I'd met was my American friend Cynthia in Barcelona. I had learned about this profession through her when it was unheard of yet in Turkey. Her financial advice had helped me overcome some weaknesses I experienced with my clients while I was practicing architecture in Barcelona. Life coaches cannot give you what you want in life but they can help you find the keys to unlock the doors to your aspirations. Our sessions with Paul benefited me a great deal. In a way, he helped me find my way when I was lost. They say a good beginning is half the battle. The guidance of the life coach helped me take that first step I'd been hesitating to take.

My brother Can had been wishing to open a café in Tekirdağ for a long time and looking for a suitable place. He had finally found and bought a run-down, three-story building in the town center and wanted me to do the architectural project for the renovation and undertake the interior decoration. It was a great opportunity for me. Work would distract me and creating something would make me feel productive again. Losses and failures I'd suffered made me feel as if I was never going to succeed in life. This was going to pass and all would be well again in a while but I struggled with this feeling of having hit rock bottom for a long time...

An Accident & an Experience with a Psychotherapist

I decided to see the psychotherapist recommended by the hospital to find answers to the questions I'd been constantly asking myself since my loss and to stop blaming myself. I felt much relieved even after the very first session. I think it worked so fast because I both believed it would and could open up easily. It was good to hear the opinion of an outsider, especially if that outsider was an expert on the troubles of women dealing with the loss of a child. Was I never to have a child like a normal woman? When I told him of how I blamed myself and struggled with feelings of inadequacy, he said, "I know so many women who went through the same things as you, you are not alone and what you feel is totally normal. I have a patient who lost her baby a few days after the birth; she is seven months pregnant now. She has a phobia for postpartum period that we work at overcoming." Then he added, "Don't be afraid to try again."

It felt good to hear of others who'd had the same or similar experiences, it helped me see myself as a normal woman again. When I asked him what I could do to forget about them, he told me I shouldn't try to forget. "They are part of your life. They've been with you for a while but they are not there any longer. Don't try to exclude them from your life; that would be a mistake. They are your babies. Give them names. Imagine you've buried them, visualize them resting in peace. Go visit them if you need to... in your mind or in real life." I did as I was told. I named them with the names I had hoped to call them, I imagined they were buried under the large pine tree in the garden of the hospital. I pictured them in heaven, thinking of me. I shared this fantasy with my husband. Our twins that we'd been trying to forget now became a part of our life, they were our babies who had been with us for a while. Thinking this way, however unbelievable it may sound, strangely alleviated my pain.

One day, as I was driving to an appointment, a car just overtook from my right side and took a U-turn at the junction ahead. Obviously the driver, a woman, was in a hurry to get somewhere, and she apparently was somewhat oblivious of the rules of the road, considering the way she passed me from the wrong side. I slammed on the brakes with my fast reflexes honed in the crazy

Istanbul traffic yet couldn't avoid scratching the car. The driver who overtook was a hundred percent to blame. I got out of the car and told her calmly that she was at fault. Thinking I was going to make her pay for all the damage, she looked at me with eyes begging for mercy. When I told her I forgave her she just stared, unable to believe her ears. It was most probably the first time she'd ever come across such a reaction from a stranger in Belgium. This accident was nothing compared to the loss I'd incurred two months ago, which was probably why I was so calm. In my mind, I could hear a song playing; Candan Erçetin's Yalan, of which words translate roughly as "Everything on earth is a lie, but death."

Belgians are extremely meticulous, and irritable, about their cars. I knew that very well as I'd had to deal with it before. I could have had the owner of the car who'd hit mine pay for all the damage. One day when we'd just moved to Brussels, we'd been shopping in Ikea and I'd come back to the parking lot with all the packages, ready to place them in the car, so I had to open the car door wide. I judged by eye the distance between our car and the one parked next to us. I was very careful, but the driver of the other car jumped out furiously and accused me of scratching his car without even checking it. He insisted that we had damaged his car. I was mad, either we were blind or he was hallucinating, as there was not a scratch to be seen. Obviously he was looking to have his car painted at somebody else's expense, and it was his lucky day as he had come across foreigners. He must have seen our plate number because we still drove under a Spanish plate. We weren't able to come to terms with the man as he only spoke Dutch and very little English and he didn't seem willing to come to terms with us anyway. The dispute grew more serious. He was obviously determined to make us pay for his car door. He called the police, the officers who came did only speak Dutch like him and just bought whatever he said. Being foreigners, we were at a disadvantage from the start, we could see there was no way we could reconcile no matter what we did. We were new in the country and didn't know the laws, we felt very inexperienced. We just listened to them talk between themselves without uttering a word and without understanding any of it. The police officers inspected the car door at length, and recorded the incident, even though, I felt, they couldn't quite wrap their heads around it. We left the spot grumbling about this mean man who had ruined our Ikea day and wondering whether we would end up having to pay for an imaginary damage. As we hoped, we didn't hear of this any further and it remained in our memory as a "Welcome to Brussels" experience.

My brother Can needed me and we had to start the project as soon as possible. So I went to Tekirdağ for 10 days, leaving my husband alone. I'd visited the hospital psychotherapist only twice, after which he must have thought I didn't need any more sessions as he'd told me I could stop seeing him. I could also see the progress I'd made. I was feeling a lot more normal. I was still carrying 13 of the 20 pounds I'd gained during pregnancy. All the fat reserve I'd put on was still there. And my breasts were filled with milk, which really affected me. A long time after the end of my pregnancy, seeing them enlarged as they were every time I looked in the mirror kept reminding me of my loss. In the hospital, I'd been given a medicine to stop milk production after the delivery, but during the first nights and days my breasts just released milk on their own, and I couldn't help crying when I saw my nightgown soaked with milk. Fortunately, the drug eventually took effect and milk release stopped after the second day but the weeping took a lot longer to cease...

One Day...

'One day,' I often thought, wondering whether I too would be a mother one day... When was that day to come? I asked myself this so many times, I virtually lived with the question. I wanted that baby so badly! While I was looking ahead, far ahead in the future, my dream was about to come true a lot sooner. My beautiful Istanbul was waiting for me with a generous gift...

4

Brussels II

It was a nice and warm spring morning in May 2006. The doorbell rang. It was the mailman. I went down and checked the mailbox, to find a wedding invitation. It was great news, my dear friend Rebi was getting married to her true love, Ata!

I couldn't miss that wedding! We bought tickets with Brussels Airlines and arranged our work to fly to Istanbul for the wedding that was to take place on the 4th of June. I couldn't possibly miss the chance of being with my friend on that great day, and it would also give me the opportunity to see my parents. Furthermore, June is a lovely time of the year, the days are long, the nights are happy, so it would be a nice short break for us. We were fed up with rain in Brussels, it would do us good to get in the mood for summer. There was a long way to go till August, when the Europeans usually took their holidays, which we did too (although we didn't like it), because the European Commission and Parliament, and many factories closed in August and therefore my husband, who worked in a bank, was less busy.

We hadn't been to Turkey since we lost the twins. I knew it would upset me to have to tell everyone the story over and over again but maybe it might find relief in pouring my heart out. The psychotherapist of the hospital in Brussels insisted that I should face it and should not try to forget them, saying they were a part of my life. He also advised, "Don't start trying to conceive again for a while, give yourself time, you need to recover both physically and mentally and relax." I normally liked to stick to experts' advice but when I set my mind on something I wouldn't let anything stop me. So I decided to follow my inner voice instead of the therapist's advice. It wasn't for me to rest, I found it taxing. So I went back to the university hospital three months after I lost the twins, told the doctor I was feeling well and said resolutely, "Let's do it!" And we were ready to try artificial insemination for the second time before our trip to Turkey.

✦

My quadruple pregnancy and the high dose hormone shots I'd been given last time had scared me. I wasn't going to let this happen again. The doctors were quite cautious too, this time, and gave me lower doses of hormone supplements. The procedure was the same as in our first try: Sonograms starting on the 11th day of my cycle and repeating every other day, waiting for the eggs to reach the adequate size for fertilization. Finally, they were large enough on the 16th day, and I went to the laboratory to have the shot to stimulate their release. We were now familiar with the procedure as it was our second time around. As we knew what to expect we were quite relaxed, taking it lightly. We went to the hospital early, around 8 o'clock in the morning.

While I sat leafing through magazines in the reception area, my husband was shown in that infamous little room. When he came out, he told me bashfully about the porn magazines and videos in the room and we giggled like teenagers, drawing astonished stares from the other patients waiting gravely and stressfully. They seemed to be saying, "We are here for a serious business, what's with those two?" We had to wait another two hours while the sperm was "washed and prepared" like veggies to go into a stew, following which I was admitted to the big room. It was a technical procedure but my husband and I tried to make it a sweet moment, he sat near me and held my hand through the insemination procedure, which took only a few minutes. The nurse told me to keep my lying position for another 5 to 10 minutes but I just remained on the chair for almost half an hour to allow the sperm to swim to their destination. As Cosimo was there, caressing my hair, I didn't mind waiting.

The nurse finally had to ask us to leave, saying another patient was soon to be admitted in the room and that I'd had enough rest. We were used to the aloofness of the hospital staff, we didn't care. Cosimo couldn't help joking as we left the room: "I hope we don't end up having a black baby!" and we giggled. We were so accustomed to the ways of the hospital that nothing got to us anymore. In the car, I reclined my seat all the way, Cosimo started the car and turned on the radio, a singer with a soft voice was singing a Blues song. We went into the tunnel connecting the hospital to our home, we stared into each other's eyes in the darkness and wished for luck. It was obvious we both had the same thing in mind, even if we didn't say it out loud: we wanted that baby soooo much!

Failures

Sad news were awaiting us in Turkey. Our dog Fındık, who had been guarding our summer house, had been poisoned. It was a mild tempered creature, who'd never been a nuisance to anyone. Who could have ruthlessly slain that good dog! We suspected the neighbors but we couldn't blame anyone as there were no witnesses. My parents hadn't wished to give me the bad news on the phone and waited for me to come home. It was the first time in years I saw my father that sad, he was out of spirits for days. Fındık was his friend, his walking companion. A few days later, he came with a cardboard box in hand, with the cutest little puppy in it. A friend of his who saw how miserable he was had given him one of the newborn puppies of his dog. I fell in love with the tiny puppy with its black hair, black eyes and white patches on its ears and throat as soon as I saw it. I wanted to kiss it and nuzzle it but it was so scared, so insecure, so timid... As I wasn't a mother yet, I couldn't understand how vulnerable a month-old puppy was. It needed its mother more than anything.

The first night, we made him a spot out in the balcony. We gave him some milk and laid him on soft cushions. In the middle of the night, I woke up with a noise like a baby crying. Still sleepy, I ran to the noise, not knowing what it was, to see it was our little guest, who'd wandered out of his kennel and was shaking and looking at me with sad, pleading eyes. I couldn't resist it, I had to take it in to our room. With Cosimo, we made it a place on the foot of the bed and it went to sleep comfortably after watching us for a while. It was obviously scared to be alone. After some time, it woke up, came to me wagging its little tail and looking at me anxiously. I tried to comfort him to no avail and couldn't understand what it wanted until it went to a corner and peed. Poor little one, it slept in peace with us that night. I took it to its kennel in the balcony early in the morning, before my mother saw it in the bedroom. Unfortunately, it wasn't eating much and growing weaker from day to day. We didn't know what to do. We took it to the vet, who gave us some vitamin supplements. It was too young to get a vaccine yet. It would be better off with its mother but I was unable to figure it out then. The poor little puppy died a few days later, maybe because it didn't nurse long enough, or maybe because it was weak from the beginning, its little body couldn't handle it.

This shook me deeply. I had lost pets before but obviously I was very sensitive and vulnerable at that time. Failures made me feel inadequate. 'Nur, you can't even take care of a puppy, no wonder you can't have a baby,' I kept telling myself, and blaming myself harshly. People always said I was motherly but apparently it was only how I looked and it wasn't enough; what good was it to look the part if I couldn't play it.

The Wedding

We'd been staying at my parents' summer house in Tekirdağ for a few days, swimming and getting tan. We were in good shape and ready for the wedding. But on the morning of the wedding, I woke up with a nasty surprise. My period, which was a few days late, making me wonder if we'd done it, had arrived. What a disappointment it was! We hadn't got there, it hadn't worked! The first time we'd tried artificial insemination I'd conceived straight away – even though it had been for nothing. Why had we failed this time? Was I getting older and my ovulation diminishing? Was I too late to be a mom? I already had trouble carrying a pregnancy to term, was I to have trouble getting pregnant (and despite therapy!) now? If artificial insemination didn't work, should we try IVF? When I broke the bad news to my husband, he was upset and his face fell.

We were hardly in the mood for a wedding. I put on my white ensemble embroidered with pink blossoms (similar to the style that Audrey Hepburn used to wear), that I was looking forward to wearing to the wedding, and I put on my make-up carelessly. We started heading to wedding in Istanbul from Tekirdağ. We didn't talk much during the two hour drive, almost as if we were afraid to talk about it. The view of the Bosphorus cheered us a little bit. It was a beautiful summer evening in early June. We were in Ulus 29, Istanbul, where Rebi and Ata's wedding was to take place. I remembered our wedding, which was one of the happiest moments in my life. The legal ceremony had taken place here in Ulus 29, with a view on the Bosphorus. Even though it was an autumn night the weather was summer-mild, luckily for us. This place is the perfect venue for a wedding with its unique view of the Bosphorus, its delightful decoration designed by Zeynep Fadıllıoğlu down to the finest detail, its excellent cuisine and impeccable service; there is no place like it, very classy, although a little expensive. Every time I prepare an Istanbul tour guide for my friends visiting the city I make a point of telling them not to leave Istanbul without having dinner in Ulus 29.

I inhaled the refreshing Bosphorus air and tried to smile. My dear friend was elated tonight, I shouldn't be unhappy, or at least

I should conceal it and smile for her. Seeing Cosimo's long face reminded me of what I tried to forget, making me sulk too. It was so hard to try and look happy after all we'd been through for years to have a baby...

We sipped our delicious cocktails in the warm breeze, catching up with old friends. We enjoyed the view with my husband, just like we did in our own wedding night, him standing behind me with his arms around me. He was holding me so tight, so lovingly, that he seemed to say "Hang in there, darling, we must be strong, we must not lose heart in face of these failures!" We didn't talk, we just listened to each other's breathing and to the sound of Istanbul at night. Suddenly we heard a roar of applause: the bride and groom were coming in. When I saw them coming through the door, I couldn't keep my tears from rolling down my cheeks, joy and sadness mixed and mingled in those tears. I was so happy for Rebi...

Rebi looked so beautiful and happy! She was wearing a gorgeous bridal gown similar to that of a Greek goddess, with a pleated skirt, that she carried so handsomely with her tall, gracious figure. Her long, black hair cascaded down her shoulders in waves, she was wearing soft make-up on her lightly tanned face. She was a lovely summer bride.

The ceremony table was placed just like it was at our wedding, with the bride and groom facing the guests and their back to the Bosphorus. From our point of view, the bride and groom over a lovely backdrop of Bosphorus vista looked like the very image of eternal happiness and love. Then the girls made a circle with the bride in the middle and we took it in turns to dance with her. When it was my turn, we hugged each other tightly, I could feel how happy and excited she was when I held her. And Ata, the groom, was beaming with happiness all night. It was almost impossible to talk under the loud music, Rebi approached my ear to say, "I'm sooo happy, Nurcuk."*

"I know," I replied, "and I'm happy for you." When she said, "I have another great reason to be happy, I'm pregnant," we both started to weep for joy. We hugged and kissed again. The onlookers couldn't understand the reason for our excitement and went on with their dancing. Oh, what I wouldn't give to be pregnant like her. All of the sudden, I remembered the disappointment of the morning and was filled with sadness. I couldn't possibly tell Rebi of my setback on the night of her wedding of all nights, so I tried to avoid her eyes and did my best to not let my sorrow show.

I just couldn't help it, once more, my mind was swarming with dark thoughts, the same question as ever: "Shall I ever have a baby?" Tears kept swelling in my eyes, still wet from crying, as I asked myself that question over and over again. I watched the Bosphorus with my teary eyes. The lights were dancing. Istanbul, at night, made me even more sad.

Confession in the Swiss Hotel

Cosimo had to go back to work in Brussels in the morning, but I could see his reluctance. He didn't like to fly back home alone after our holiday and he always found it hard to leave me and Istanbul. He didn't say anything, but I knew from the way he looked, he was in low spirits. We hugged tight as if to say to one another,

---

* Turkish diminutive for Nur.

"We failed again, so what, we've got each other." I wanted to stay on a few more days to do a few odd jobs but it broke my heart to see him like that. We were going to be away from each other only for a few days, and although we'd been married for six years, we couldn't bear to be apart. Waving goodbye, I told myself I was a lucky woman to have him.

Rebi and Ata had spent their wedding night at the Swiss Hotel. That morning, she called me and invited me over for coffee. After dropping Cosimo at the airport, I drove to the hotel and Rebi and I sank in the comfortable sofas in the lobby. We commented about the wedding night over a cup of coffee. "What an energetic bride you are," I said to her. "The bride is usually exhausted after the wedding, but you look just fine, and you are pregnant, too!" Rebi was always a super active girl who could do fifty different things in one day and expecting hadn't changed that. She was looking at my face with searching eyes and she could tell something was wrong, even though I tried not to let it on. I really needed to talk since yesterday but I couldn't possibly talk to Cosimo as he was even more upset than I; and I didn't want to tell my mother over the phone (all she would say would be "Don't worry, my darling girl, you will have a child," anyway), so I really needed to talk to someone and vent my feelings.

I told Rebi of what happened and my eyes were filled with tears. How could a woman who'd got pregnant just like that, without even trying, understand how I felt, but she was sorry to see me cry and tried to comfort me, to give me some advice. I envied her for having gotten pregnant so easily, maybe I was even a little jealous of her. I was cross with myself because I had to be happy for her, which I was, for sure. Rebi deserved a happy marriage and a happy home with a baby. I didn't want to upset her any more, and Ata had missed his wife and came down to join us anyway. I left the newlyweds alone in the hotel and went to one of Istanbul's giant malls to distract myself from my depressing thoughts. I amused myself with window shopping and bought some trinkets to reward myself. I met a friend of mine for tea in the afternoon, and she filled me in on the country news and the latest gossip. I didn't feel as upset as I was before about what had happened the other day anymore, and I didn't feel I had failed, I felt better.

Decision Day

The next morning, I jumped out of bed excitedly. My period was a window of opportunity for me. Why shouldn't I try again? I decided to see the doctor without delay. My instincts told me to try again. I was psychologically very motivated. Spending the last two days with Rebi had made me forget my hopelessness and find my desire to be a mom once more.

Not that I ever lost that desire, but sometimes the disappointments I went through made me waver and think that maybe I wasn't cut out to be a mother. But now I had shaken that pessimistic mood off and felt totally ready for the wearisome treatment ahead. I wanted to call my doctor in Brussels straight away but it was too early to call. I went to wake my brother Can up. "Wake up, little brother. Let's go to that famous breakfast place of ours and feast on honey and cream!" My brother, who liked to sleep on till late in the morning looked at me with sleepy eyes, wondering why we were in a hurry to go to eat. Breakfast was only a way for me to distract myself until the time I could talk to my doctor and clarify my decision.

I reached my doctor with some difficulty. I told him our last attempt had failed and I wanted to try again, if it was alright. I also told him I was in Turkey and asked if I could start treatment in a fertility center here in Istanbul and go on with them when I was back in Brussels. I was anxious for a favorable answer and jumped for joy when he said, "Sure, it's perfectly fine. Just call us as soon as you get back so we can proceed as necessary." I called my gynecologist in Istanbul immediately to make an appointment.

A friend of mine who suffered of lazy ovaries like me and whose opinion I trusted had told me about her gynecologist in Istanbul. She had gone through infertility treatment, and had given birth to healthy twins, one boy and one girl. Her doctor, Dr. Aret Kamar, was a young, successful gynecologist, well known in fertility treatment and very popular among his patients. He had an IVF center that he had established single handedly, where he treated people from all over Turkey and from all socio-economic groups, who came to see him for various problems. He didn't give IVF treatment to everyone, this wasn't just a 'business' to him; he really cared. As soon as I stepped in through the door, I was filled with confidence, which was doubled when I met the Dr. Aret. I was thankful to my friend for telling me about him. I believed I'd found the right doctor this time. He listened carefully to my medical history with his two assistants, taking notes. Towards the end of my narrative my voice started breaking and my eyes were filled with tears, as it happened every time I had to talk about this. (I don't know if I could tell my story with the same surge of sentimentality now but before I had children, I couldn't help tears rolling down my cheeks every time I told it; now I only feel tears swell in my eyes.

I hated to cry in front of doctors, nurses, and staff that I'd never met before, and tried in vain to compose myself and tell my story soberly. No matter what I did, I ended up crying in front of maybe a hundred health care professionals. The doctor comforted me with kind words and told me he thought we could start treatment as I was menstruating. "Don't worry, we'll give you a low dose of hormones. Let's start tomorrow without delay," he says as he opens an oblong box that looks like a pen case, with a tiny syringe holding 500 ml of a hormone supplement. I was to give myself a dose of a 100 ml every day with a shot on the belly. Although I was frightened of shots, I was able to do it as the needle was really short and thin, looking almost like a mechanical pencil tip. I was amazed at myself, normally I wouldn't even be able to watch someone or myself having an injection but now I could give myself an injection, it was unbelievable what you could do to have a baby!

Although there was no pregnancy in sight yet, Dr. Aret gave me a prescription with the drugs I was supposed to take during pregnancy. I was pleased. It was good to have a doctor who thought ahead. Normally, one would start to take folic acid supplements* a few months before getting pregnant. I hadn't started as I had no intention, or hope, of trying again, but Dr. Aret said it was not too late. Statistically, how many women get pregnant exactly when

---

* You have to take folic acid supplements, tiny pills of great merit, which can affect the whole life of your baby to be born, before you get pregnant. The deficiency of folic acid may cause spinal malformation in the baby.

they plan to or how many start using folic acid on time, anyway? Also, I'd been using it four months ago, when I was pregnant, so I must still have some in my system. I'd been given so many pills and shots before and during pregnancy that I couldn't even remember the names.

Besides folic acid and multi vitamin supplements, Dr. Aret prescribed baby Aspirin as well, to thin the blood, as he believes it prevents miscarriages... Baby Aspirin is Aspirin with a very low dosage, it tastes good too! This must be the nicest medicine I've taken during all my pregnancies so far. I'd never have thought I would be taking the little pink pills I used to take when I was a child while I'm trying to have a baby. Blood clotting is one of the reasons causing miscarriages, so I also have a daily shot of Fragmin, a drug given to cardiovascular patients with clotting problems. (I still remember the burn and the bruise marks caused by those shots in every inch of my belly. You couldn't see the skin around my waist! The desire to keep that baby in your womb can make you do anything!) And I am to start on Progestin as soon as my pregnancy is confirmed. Dr. Aret says it is very important and that it will probably be emphasized by my doctor in Brussels too.

The Return & the Waiting

I'm at the exit gate in Brussels Airport, Cosimo mi amore is there, waiting for me. We've only been separated for six days but since we are not used to it we find it hard to bear. "Our home is unbearable without you," he says, "and I hate being alone at home after a holiday." Although I don't want to raise his hopes unnecessarily, I'm too excited to keep it a secret. "This time it was for a good reason!" I tell him that I've started treatment in Istanbul. We drive home chirping cheerfully. Are we the same couple who was almost in mourning last Sunday? I tell him of the week I spent away from him in full detail. He can feel how much I trust my new doctor, he is amazed but also glad that I'm so enthusiastic. I don't have anything to lose any more, I've dealt with such difficulties that it's almost a part of my life to be prepared for that tedious process that's awaiting us...

I make my first appointment back in Brussels and the adventure starts all over again on the 11th day of my cycle. The eggs finally reached the required size on the 19th day. Now they will be released, helped with a shot, and then my darling husband will give his precious sperm, we will make our usual jokes of African, Chinese, Japanese babies to cheer ourselves up, then I will be admitted in the AI room while the sperm will be "washed and prepared" in for the big ritual...

On day-D, auditors from Italy visit the bank where my spouse is working. He is very nervous, anxious to get back to work and prepare for the audit. I tell him he needn't wait for another two hours to stay with me during the insemination, I don't mind driving. I'm used to it now, I don't fret about it like I used to do. Cosimo goes to his meeting, I pass the time looking through the magazines. Finally, the long awaited moment... As it's my third time around, I don't worry anymore, after the insemination I lie on the operation chair for 10 minutes only, whereas I used remain there much longer in the previous times, and then I leave the hospital walking calmly. I get into the car and drive into the darkness of the famous tunnel crossing the city. I am, of course, nervous and excited but this time I'm a little more relaxed and I'm very hopeful, as always. As the car dives into the darkness of the tunnel, I dive into my never-ending dreams of having a baby.

We are called in for a blood test in two weeks. My hormone levels will be checked and they will tell us whether or not I'm pregnant. I'm very excited but prepared to face any result, be it positive or negative; if the test result turns out to be negative I'll not worry and try to think positive – even though I don't quite know how. My husband and I have given our word to each other, we will not give up!

Best News Ever!

I'm waiting for the call from the hospital, jumping every time the phone rings. And finally the long awaited call: "Congratulations, you are pregnant!" Oh my God, how it's nice to hear! It's the sentence every woman who wants a baby is dying to hear...

The first few days, I feel confused. For one thing, I cannot believe I'm pregnant. Second, I'm troubled with questions and worries, considering what I've been through in the past. What am I to do now? Will I be able to have a healthy pregnancy? Will I be able to go through the first trimester safe and sound? And the fifth month? And all through to the end of my pregnancy, and hold my baby in my arms, finally?

The morning sickness I'd experienced in all my previous pregnancies comes troubling me again. I already have to take a handful of pills and get shots in the belly every day, hours of nausea on top of it is just too much, I spend my whole day between the kitchen and the bathroom. You go to the kitchen, open the fridge and stare inside, not knowing what it is you are looking for. Nothing looks appetizing, or, nothing looks as if it could quell your nausea. You eat a bread stick, which at first seems to calm your stomach but it's unavoidable to throw up eventually, you run to the bathroom and hug the toilet bowl... After you turn totally inside out, morning sickness finally passes, giving way to pregnancy reflux, and heartburn this time. The level of progestogen increases during pregnancy, slowing down bowel movements, and may cause constipation. I get my share of that too and I have to sit on the toilet for hours. So basically, the bathroom is my new living quarters. They say not every pregnancy is the same but for me it follows the same typical pattern every time. All the hormones in my body go wild and hit me.

I'm not complaining, just telling my husband of my 'troubles' from time to time to steal more attention, that's all. In truth, experiencing all these pregnancy symptoms makes me extremely happy, it feels like a confirmation of my situation and it's the best antidote to my phobia of miscarriage. I love being pregnant! I love nausea, oversensitivity to tastes and smells, heartburn, vomiting, and dizziness! I love constipation, back pain, leg cramps and varicose veins, stuffy nose, breathlessness, indigestion, incontinence, waking up several times during the night to go to the bathroom, not getting any sleep, and the white patches all over my body! I am prepared to face everything that can happen to me, because, although I may not be a seasoned mom, I'm a seasoned expectant mom, as weird and ironic as it may sound. I'm an expert on pregnancy as I've been reading about it all through my pregnancies. Inevitably, you forget some of it and can't help asking your doctor strange questions.

When I was pregnant, I used to write down my questions in

a notepad I always carried with me, browse through them before my appointments and cross over the ones I'd found the answers to. Today we can access information so quickly and effectively thanks to the Internet, books, and media! But even when we've found our answers on a different source, we still want to ask our doctor to be sure; the words of a doctor whom we trust is above everything else we may hear or read. We, women, ask our ob-gyn countless questions, but my questions were quite different from the ones frequently asked. I could usually find the answers to the most typical questions in other sources and kept the unusual ones for my doctor. When I look through my old pregnancy notebooks now, I see so many questions I wrote down to ask, some of which I now find unnecessary and some very useful. Here are some of the questions I asked my doctors in different countries: In Turkey: "Can I eat shrimp, fish, Tulum cheese (goat cheese), salami, sausages, sujuk, or salad? Can I drink herbal teas? Can I have a massage, go in the sauna, have a bath, ride a boat, or swim in Marmara Sea?" In Spain, some questions still remain, while I have some new ones: For example, "Can I swim in Barcelona? What is safe to eat in a seafood heaven such as Spain? Can I eat ham?" In Belgium, famous for its mussels and steak tartar (made of raw beef), I had to know if I could eat these. And, when everybody was savoring the famous Belgian beers I apparently wanted to join in the fun and asked, "Can I at least drink non-alcoholic beer?" And exercise was an issue as well: "Can I work out regularly? Can I do other popular exercises such as aqua-yoga or kinetherapy to help labor?" And the list goes on...

An Italian Wedding

I love summer weddings and this summer has lots of them. This time, it's my sister-in-law who's getting married and we're going to Italy. The trip worries me a little and I hesitate as I'm scared of traveling while expecting since I had lost the twins right after the trip to Barcelona, which may have been just a coincidence but I have blamed myself so much afterwards. I really want to be there to share my sister-in-law's happiness and I'm not even two months along yet, so the fetus is too small to be affected from external influences. I ask the doctor whether the plane trip might be dangerous. I can't help it, I'm scared!

The white ensemble I've worn to Rebi's wedding is already too tight! I always gain at least 7 pounds in the first trimester of my pregnancies, and this time is no exception: four pounds and a half in two months! The suit was snug to start with, now that I've gained weight it hugs my form so tightly that the stiches might break. I browse through my wardrobe to find something I can wear to the wedding. All the suits and dresses that fit are in dark colors. I dislike going shopping especially for something to wear on a special occasion, so I pick one of the dark dresses to wear in the heat of summer, but I'm grateful anyway to find something that fits. Everything is ready, we are going to Italy, and not just for the wedding, it's going to be a wonderful break!

My dear sister-in-law has captured my heart once more by making a reservation for us in a spa hotel in Abano Terme, a thermal resort up on a hill near Padua, where the wedding is to take place. I used to go to Gönen Thermal Resort in Turkey every year with my grandparents, which is probably why I love spas. The hotels were not that fancy then, of course, usually only visited for therapeutic purposes. My grandparents used to like to spend a couple of weeks there, following their doctors' advice. Today the spa hotels have evolved into relaxation and beauty centers, like the one in Padua where we are staying. The hotel, which has a spa, offers endless choices of physiotherapy, including kinesitherapy, hydrokinesitherapy, and physiokinesitheraly, ranging from Ayurveda to Reiki, Reflexology, Shiatsu and Watsu... Expecting mothers have to avoid excessive heat, so I stay away from the thermal pool, which I don't fancy anyway, the weather being so hot. I confine myself to Reflexology foot massage, not advised against during pregnancy. The mountain air is good for me, even though I cannot benefit from the thermal waters. I inhale the clean, fresh air, praying for my baby to be alright.

Apparently, I'm not to rest easy! The morning before the wedding I wake up to a nasty surprise: there is a red spot in my underwear! I know that in some pregnancies light spotting may be seen during the first trimester and it may be alright, but I can't help worrying. I'm seized by the fear of miscarriage. In my second pregnancy, I'd had some light bleeding a few days before the miscarriage, which had given way to a phobia and I'd been checking my underwear obsessively every time I went to the toilet.

"Shall I ever have an uneventful and untroubled pregnancy?" I murmur to myself and I'm stuck in the bathroom of our hotel suite. I keep thinking whether I've done anything wrong during the last few days or whether there is something wrong with my pregnancy. My doubts converge on the plane trip and the reflexology massage. "You've done it again, Nur," I scold myself, "why can't you just stay put," although I know the spotting has nothing to do with any of this. I often keep things to myself as I don't want to worry my husband unnecessarily; I can handle my own panic but I cannot deal with his at the same time. I don't want to alarm him, especially on this very day where his beloved sister is getting married. There isn't anything to be done at this moment anyway, even if there's something wrong. I decide to call my doctor in Turkey, who tells me I shouldn't worry and that the spotting has probably nothing to do with the embryo and is likely a blood discharge from the womb, and advises me to go to the hospital if I feel any pain. Talking to him comforts me a little and I try to think positively and not to blame myself.

Abano, the land of thermal spas, on an emerald green hill... It's July, the hottest month in this region and the place is burning hot. The wedding ceremony takes place in a pretty little mountain church, followed by a cocktail party in the gardens of a historical villa at the foot of the hill. Then there is the wedding dinner and the party goes on till after midnight. It's a lovely wedding and I have a great time with my Italian in-laws, chatting, laughing, and dancing. I even forget all my concerns about my pregnancy for a few hours.[*]

*My article that appeared in my column Hola Barcelona! In Elele magazine, September 2006: An Italian Wedding.

Sorellina; that is my dear sister-in-law is getting married! The groom is a Veneto, from Venice, and the wedding is to take place in Padua, Italy... I've never been to an Italian wedding before even though I'm married to an Italian, our wedding took place in Istanbul, which makes it more of a Turkish wedding with a lot of guests from Italy. Actually, the contemporary weddings today, except traditional weddings, are the same all over the world, the only difference in Catholic countries being the ceremony being performed in a church. The rest is basically the same everywhere; the wedding dinner is eaten on large, round tables where the guests are seated in groups, there is either a band or a DJ playing music, a photographer going around, flashing constantly, while the bride and groom go around the tables, hugging and kissing each guest and posing for their picture to be taken. Then comes the wedding cake (the larger the better) on a wheeled table. The bride and groom slice through it together with a huge knife that looks like a sword. Then they feed each other some cake and sip some Champagne with their arms entwined like the sprigs of a vine. The first dance is set to a romantic song. Then, as the elderly start leaving, the party mood gradually rises, the music gets livelier and louder, popular songs are played and everyone dances. Single men ask single women to dance. The bride throws her bouquet, and her single friends who wish to get married soon try to catch it. The bride and groom look forward to seeing the last of the guests leave, and at the end of the night sink into their bed, too tired to enjoy any romance.

As most of the young couples coming from modern families have been together for some time before getting married, the wedding night has lost its importance. In the wedding in Italy, I noticed a few fancy rituals different from ours in Turkey, for example, a week or so before the wedding, humorous wedding notices are hung on the neighbors' doors; the wedding gifts are sent to the couple's house about a month before the wedding as it makes furnishing easier and giving jewelry to the bride and groom on the wedding is not common; the bride and groom are not allowed to see one another for a night and a day before the wedding, the bride is taken into the church and 'given' to the groom by her father; one of the couple's family members of friends reads a poem or a composition he or she has written about them; rice is thrown on *the bride and groom as they emerge from the church as a symbol of prosperity and fertility; at the end of the reception the groom removes the bride's garter and tosses it to the single man and the one to catch it is believed to be the first marry... My sister-in-law Ivana, whom I call sorellina, which means little sister in Italian, was pregnant three years after her wedding, at the age of 35, after trying to conceive for over a year, but without having to resort to fertility treatment. The doctors had to perform a lot of test and examinations before they could find out she had a cyst and treated it. She had nine months of a trouble-free pregnancy followed by a hard labor, but forgot about it all when she saw her beautiful Tomaso!*

The First Prenatal Appointment

It's the seventh week of my pregnancy and the time for my first prenatal appointment. We hear the embryo's heartbeat, a moment that moves me every time. It's a great feeling to create a living being, to carry it inside you. All I want at this moment is for this baby to be healthy, to grow safe and sound in my womb, and to be born. On one hand, the doubts: "Am I going to make it this time?" On the other, the wishes: "Come on, baby, don't let me down! I want you more than anything, I want to be your mom, please let me." Once you've hit rock bottom maybe you lose your fears, or you learn to live with them. I don't know which it is, but all I know is that: at that moment when I'm listening to that heartbeat inside me, I don't want to think about anything else. I promise myself to enjoy every moment of my pregnancy, every moment with my baby, without obsessing about tomorrow...

❧

There are two dreadful obstacles ahead of me: the first trimester and then the 20th week. There are different theories explaining the reasons for my two previous miscarriages, but the real reason remains to be known for sure. Although I want to enjoy my pregnancy thoroughly I can't shake off my fears. I keep thinking that I could do anything to have a safe pregnancy. I'm normally of an optimistic nature; I don't make a big issue of the problems I encounter. I am solution-oriented and I like to see the good part in everything, but when pregnancy and babies are involved I am not myself anymore. I become pessimistic and anxious. I cannot think straight. I feel all the misfortunes find me of all people and I despair. I get a yeast infection once or twice a year, that I treat easily with antifungal cream, but when I'm pregnant I fuss about it so much it's unbelievable! I cannot sleep, I agonize, I worry about it reaching the womb through the vagina and hurting the baby somehow. My doctor has told me not to read too much on the Internet and confuse myself, but I cannot stop. I keep coming up with questions that have to Google and after a while I get exhausted in front of the computer screen and end up reading everything that's ever been written about it!

Row, Row, Row Your Boat...

It's the same every time I'm pregnant, I'm both elated and anxious at the same time. One minute I'm over the moon, the next I'm down. It's almost a love-hate relationship in itself. As I'm keen on my freedom I find it irritating to be constrained, which I can only bear thanks to my love for the baby. But what I find hardest to bear is the constant feeling of guilt, feeling as if I'm not fulfilling my responsibilities towards the baby I'm carrying. I don't know what pregnancy brings after the first five months as I've never gone further, and I'm hoping this anxiousness won't continue until the end of the pregnancy, hoping I can relax and enjoy my baby growing in my belly.

Our friends Paola and Michel, a sociable couple with whom we along very well and take part in many activities together like spending their weekends doing sports. Before I got pregnant, as we'd been planning on doing canoeing together for some time, they found a class we could take and organized the whole thing. As soon as the weather warmed up a little, we went to the canoe club, which was very close to Brussels. I was in desperate need of new pursuits to distract myself from the painful loss of the twins. I was the best in canoeing, I could run rings around the others in the group.

Since I was used to rowing ever since I was a child, I became the instructor's pet from the first lesson. He insisted that we participate in the canoe races in Netherlands. We took a break from canoeing with the arrival of summer during which I got pregnant. When we came back to Brussels at the end of summer, with Paola's encouragement, we decided to take up our training where we'd left off and we went to the club a Saturday morning. I didn't want my husband to stop doing sports just because of me. As we didn't tell anyone I was pregnant yet I had to find some excuse to skip training, which was not that hard. I just told them I had my period and was in pain. Even though they were sorry I had to miss the fun, no one suspected anything. I watched them from a bench on the bank as they struggled with their paddles. Not that I didn't envy them, but on the other hand I was happy just to be there. I lay sprawled across the bench and enjoying my laziness. I inhale the scent of the countryside, the fresh air full of oxygen, and pray that my baby gets his share of it and grows healthily.

The Little Big Man

The infertility center on the AZ-VUB Hospital has accomplished its task and it's time for us to part with them. I'm now free to see any doctor in any hospital I wish for my prenatal care. I'm looking for a doctor that I can trust, who will follow my case closely. The Turkish, who have been living in Brussels for years, and who have become naturalized citizens talk about a Dr. Yücel Karaman. He's an ob-gyn who got his specialist's degree in Belgium, met and married a Belgian woman, and decided to settle and work in Brussels, but couldn't let go of his country. He is now a very popular doctor both in Brussels and in Istanbul. My Turkish neighbor Hülya advises me strongly to see him, telling she and her husband had a child thanks to him after trying for years and enumerating the countless miracles he's created. I have to meet him! I call straight away and make an appointment. With my darling husband who never leaves me alone the first time I'll see a doctor, we step into the office of this genius, wishing for good luck.

As we wait, sitting on the leather couches in the reception area, I examine the surroundings while Cosimo leafs through a medical journal. I'm used to the plainness of doctors' offices in Europe but I'd expect to see something different in that of a doctor from

Turkey. Apparently you don't care about decoration when you are so good at your job. Besides, how could he find the time to think about it when he worked in two different cities simultaneously! It feels good to think about trivial things to quell my nervousness.

I don't notice the passage of time as I'm distracted by these thoughts and soon it's time to go in and meet the little big man in his white coat. He looks like the ideal doctor with his warm smile and bright eyes. I tell him of my previous pregnancies and my current one, with tears in my eyes as always. He listens calmly and asks me questions. His calm comforts and assures me. He takes me on the exam chair, checks the baby, and says everything is fine, he even tells us it's probably a girl, even though it's only the fourth month of my pregnancy, with a safety margin; "I might be wrong," he says, "we'll know for sure after the tests." Cosimo and I squeeze each other's hands with emotion, our eyes filled with happiness. How everything is going well! I pray for this magic spell to go on. Dr. Karaman sits at his desk and has us sit on the chairs in front of it. "Everything looks normal," he says, "but we consider your pregnancy as critical due to your previous miscarriages, and therefore you will have to be closely monitored, which I cannot do, as I'm here only two weeks a month and in Istanbul for the other two weeks. But I'll refer you to a fellow specialist with whom I collaborate and whom I trust very much. You can be assured that he will follow your pregnancy very well," he goes on. "In the meantime, you will have your blood, urine, and HEP tests done and start taking the multivitamin supplements you need for the baby." We thank him and leave, taking the contact information of Dr. Govaerts who is to be my doctor in the future, from his assistant. We are too excited to go home, so we drive around the streets, deserted in the evening. When my excitement subsides, I realize I'm hungry and we find ourselves a nice restaurant to feast on fish. Of course, the baby is at the center of our conversation throughout the night...

A Safety Gate For My Baby

That's what I call it, a safety gate for the baby. They have to suture my cervix shut, an operation called a cervical cerclage. It's nothing new, they been using this method for a very long time. Some expectant mothers may have an incompetent cervix, which in turn may cause a miscarriage, and the condition is treated with cervical cerclage, which is basically the pursing of the cervix with a stitch. I warm to Dr. Isabelle Govaerts straight away from the first appointment, she is friendly and self-confident. She is detached, like all doctors, but kind at the same time... She greets me with the Turkish words she knows: "Merhaba, nasılsın?"* She says her husband is Turkish and she loves Turkey and the Turkish people. She examines me at length, she considers what I tell her about my pregnancy history, and, after calculating everything, she pronounces the judgment: "We will perform a precautionary cervical cerclage and close the exit temporarily so your baby won't try to come out too soon. We will suture the cervix and you will spend the rest of your pregnancy in bed rest." Cervical cerclage may seem to be a simple procedure but it is a surgical operation nonetheless and nothing like a stitch on a wounded finger. It's to be performed no later than the 13th to 14th week of my pregnancy

----

* "Hi, how are you?"

and before that, somewhere on the 10th to the 12th week I'll have the 'double test'. We make a reservation for a room at the hospital, I read and sign the consent form before the operation, which will be performed by Dr. Karaman and Dr. Govaerts, my official ob-gyn, whom I'll later call My Guardian Angel. It's important for a patient to trust their doctors. I do trust mine and I know they'll do everything in their power to make sure this baby is born healthy. I'm relaxed, I don't care about the operation or the pain or the discomfort, as long as my baby is fine and healthy!

Now, yes, we live in Europe, we are accustomed to many things, we're modern and civilized, but I have to go through a situation that I believe not even the most open minded woman on earth would consider normal. Because it's as private as it gets. I've had my facial hair removed by a male (although gay) esthetician or received massages from massage therapists before, and most of the ob-gyns I've seen so far are men, but I think this is one of the most embarrassing things you may have to do in front of a person of the opposite sex. What is it, you ask? In three words—having an enema. In more (gruesome) detail, being injected a fluid in the rectum to cause a bowel movement so all the waste material in your guts is flushed out! I'm totally not ready for something like this, either psychologically or physically! I'm caught off-guard, as vulnerable as an inpatient. This must be what they call prepping: the emptying of the bowels the night before surgery. If you are in a hospital, at the mercy of the staff, you will do as you're told, period. That's exactly what happens. A male nurse comes into my room with the necessary paraphernalia, and I do as he tells me. I don't remember having been more ashamed in my life ever...

How Do You Spend Six Months in Bed?

My doctor orders me bed rest for the rest of my pregnancy which is almost six months, saying we cannot leave anything to chance. I'm ready to do as she advises, but I just have to understand fully what bed rest exactly means, all the dos and don'ts. After all I'm a healthy expectant woman and I feel well. In fact, that's the strange thing about it, I had three miscarriages with no apparent reason. So I have to take any precautions necessary and adhere to my doctor's recommendations strictly. I ask her about what I can and cannot do in full detail. I'm allowed little trips to the kitchen and the bathroom as long as I don't stand up too long. In brief, I'm to get done with whatever I have to do and go back to bed. The white couch in the living room will be my 'base,' I'll commune with it until the end of my pregnancy. I'm told it's best if I eat my meals on the couch, in a half-reclining position. If I want to share a meal with my husband on the table, that's alright, but I have to go back to lying in the couch as soon as I finish. Also, I should shower sitting on a stool, if possible. We live in a two story apartment, with the bedrooms upstairs. It would put me in a sickly mood to spend my whole day in bed, in the bedroom, so I've picked the couch. I cannot leave home except for to go the hospital. Dr. Govaerts tells me I should forget about going to the café across the street for a cup of coffee, or popping out to buy a loaf of bread from the shop at the corner. She is very strict about the rules. She might just as well ask me to use a bedpan instead of going to the bathroom!

Of course, it's annoying for me to stay confined at home for six months and it will reduce my freedom, but I'm not sick. And, I have a great reason to put up with it, in a short while, I'll be holding my baby in my arms and forget about all this. When I think of those who are bedridden because of an ailment, spending my pregnancy at home doesn't seem so bad. It does change my lifestyle, though. At times, I feel my life is empty. Normally, I never lie down except to sleep and never sit down except to eat, bed rest is just not my thing. But I have to adapt to this new situation. I don't plan on sitting back in my large, comfy, white couch all day, I can read and write and talk to my friends if they pop in to see me.

When you're confined to bed all day, you have to have someone with you all through the day. My mother comes from Turkey to stay with me for a while, which is the greatest luxury on earth! She takes care of me like I'm a princess, but then she has her own life and I'm not comfortable with the idea that my father is left alone for a long time, so she goes back, planning to come again when her grandchild is born. My dearest husband cooks and cleans and does the laundry at night. We've had the same cleaning lady for years, Mrs. Gülten, who comes weekly to give the house a thorough cleaning. But I have to have someone to stay with me during the day.

My Mexican friend Laura recommends Celie, a Philippine lady pushing 60, but very fit and dynamic, and always smiling, that I hire as soon as I meet her. After all, I have to spend the next six months confined at home, I need to have people with positive attitudes and smiling faces around me. Celie comes to the interview with a gym bag at hand, her hair wet, and says she's coming from the swimming pool. "Way to go," I think to myself. Celie is full of respect for herself as well as for others, the only problem with her is that she cannot cook but Far Eastern dishes. Well, we are Mediterranean, we cannot have Asian food every day... So here is the solution I find: My husband is a keen cook, always fantasizing about opening a small Italian restaurant, and he's an eager follower of food literature and trends. Famous English chef Jamie Oliver is one of the chefs whose books he likes to collect. We have indeed tried many of his recipes to cook for our guests and they were all very successful, everybody liked them.

I put the books in front of Celie both so she can learn to cook new dishes and so we can try more of the recipes. She likes the idea. She's eager to learn and try new thing despite her age. And thus begins the Jamie Oliver era in our kitchen, where we try countless recipes. I choose a recipe and prepare the list of ingredients, Celie cooks and I taste. It's great entertainment while I stay at home. The story of our cook book adventure with Celie spreads around Brussels as our friends who come to visit me start talking about it. Our friends, especially those who work and like eating, but not cooking, start waiting in line to hire Celie. She has worked in several houses as a cleaning lady, a nanny, or a caregiver for elderly persons, but never as a cook before. That is until now that I've brought out the cook in her, and given her a new profession! She is happy with that, too, as she's getting offers like she never has before. She's now a cook and nanny in demand, with her phone number circulating among households in Brussels.

My social life is not bad at all, thanks to my friends who come and visit me often. I'm lucky. One of them is my truehearted Turkish friend Aylin, who, like myself, has taken her heart's advice and has come to settle in Brussels with her Swiss husband, leaving her hometown Antalya, her job and her family behind. We've met through a common American friend of ours and become great friends in no time. We live very near one another and she comes often to see and help me in so many ways. She cheers up my homebound pregnancy that I thought would be lackluster, we have long talks over a cup of tea. Sweet coincidence, she becomes pregnant as well, two months after me, so our favorite topic is pregnancy and babies. Whereas I and Cosimo are unable to pursue our many common hobbies, my confined pregnancy limits him too, but my understanding husband doesn't complain and we distract ourselves with indoor activities during that winter in Brussels.

I find our friends with whom we've lost touch for some time, call them, e-mail them, or even write them letters on pretty stationery. Cosimo brings me tulips of a different color each week, our home is turned into a flower shop. One of the nice things about living in Belgium is that you can buy your home flowers as easily as you would buy a loaf of bread from the corner shop. Thanks to the flowers, our home never misses its colors.

I get lost in the colorful world of interior decoration and fashion magazines. I decorate every corner of our home with candles, Cosimo and my mother tease me, saying our home looks like a church. When I'm alone at home, I cannot turn the natural gas fireplace on, although it's as easy as turning the tap on, as I'm not allowed to bend over, so I wait for someone to come home. I like the fire, the color, the sound, the smell of it both energize and pacify me. I love the way Cosimo strokes my belly gently while I watch the fire, sitting on my white couch. I rejoice the happiness in his eyes when he feels the 'sottomarina,' that is the submarine, move. My DJ of a husband picks the loveliest classics from his vast collection of CDs and entertains the baby and me with a musical feast. Then I indulge my palate, tasting different new dishes. Normally I have a sweet tooth but now that I'm pregnant I tend to favor savory dishes. I make sure to satisfy each one of my five senses every day that I have to spend at home, so I can keep myself and my baby happy.

My Only Entertainment: Hospital Visits!

My doctor wants to see me every 15 days, which I don't complain about, I'm glad to go as it brings some movement to my life confined between the couch and the bathroom. I'm not allowed to set step outside the door, except the 15-minute ride to the hospital when I get to look around and see what's going on outside. After we see our baby in the sonogram and hear the doctor confirm that everything is going well, Cosimo and I get back in the car to ride home, commenting on what we've seen and kissing and nuzzling each other. Naturally, I'm all teary-eyed and cry with joy.

From the seventh month onwards, I start to go to the hospital almost every week. Although my contractions haven't started yet, my doctor decides that I should take an NST every week to keep everything under control, just in case. She thinks it's a good idea to have an exam every week as some contractions are too subtle to be felt by the mother, she wants to make sure all is well. My darling husband keeps driving me to the hospital willingly every week and shows a keen interest as a caring expectant father and even has more information than I do on certain aspects of pregnancy. He's an eager Internet user and researcher anyway, and he knows in advance what I should expect on every week of my pregnancy. So he has read all about NST before we go for the first time. In the hospital, we're admitted to a small room allocated to NST only. They put two belts on my belly. I'm familiar with the procedure, as I had to take this test twice a day during the ten days I spent in the hospital for the twins. The test takes 20 minutes, during which my husband holds my hand and tries to reassure me that everything is normal, seeing the worried expression on my face, but I cannot relax before I hear the same from my doctor. The heartbeat of my son resembles the noise of the hooves of a galloping horse, it's so fast; I wonder if it's normal. I'm about to burst from anxiety when the nurse comes in, takes off the belts, gives the graphic paper a once-over and nods positively as if to say all is well, and leaves the room, saying our doctor will talk to us.

It's the routine of our life now to go to the hospital to have my contractions measured. We're used to listening to the baby's heartbeat for 20 minutes, we can't go without it for more than a week. We even call our families and have them hear it through the phone. Thankfully, everything is just fine, we are nearing the happy end without any problems in sight. I cannot believe I'm through this far, I'm so grateful. Life is beautiful, and I'm ever more relaxed as we are nearing the ninth month, which reflects both on my face and on my mood.

Hurrah, We Are Nearly There!

We are past the 32 weeks limit and both my doctor and I are relieved. We would like it for the baby to remain inside until the end of term, but we know that he has a great chance of survival if he were to be born this week. We still have about two months ahead of us, but we're already discussing labor and birth with my doctor. I tell her that C-sections are very popular in Turkey but I'm pro vaginal delivery. She has been telling me all along that I can have a normal delivery unless something unexpected comes along. I trust her, and leave everything to her. You cannot say you want this and you want that in Europe anyway, you don't have the luxury of saying you don't want to feel the pain and asking your doctor to anaesthetize you and take the baby out.

C-section is resorted to only in case it's deemed necessary. My doctor in Brussels says that 80 percent of deliveries are through C-section in Turkey and adds that it's too high a percentage. It turns out we are renowned in Europe with our C-section rates, who would have thought so!

My doctor doesn't want to leave anything to chance. If all goes well, she will go for a normal delivery but she wants to make sure my body is up for it, and asks for an MR scan. We have to see if there is a 'cephalopelvic disproportion,' in other words, whether the head of the baby is too large to pass through my pelvis. They have me lie on a gurney that they push into a narrow tunnel resembling a drawer. They give me headphones and play music at a high volume so I can stand the noise. It takes as little as little as 3 or 4 minutes but it seems like hours to me, confined in such a narrow space. The result is good, I can have a normal delivery. I didn't have any doubts about it anyway, we didn't really need the MRI, it's obvious; my pelvis and my hips are large, but my doctor just wants to be sure against any bad surprises that may come up at the last minute.

I ask my doctor's permission to go to a nearby restaurant to celebrate my husband's birthday. The place is famous and not exactly inexpensive. It's a brasserie, and naturally the chairs are

Thonet style, if it were in Turkey the clients might complain about having to sit on hard chairs when they pay so much, but here everybody is quite happy... except me!

The weight of my huge belly crushes my hips and the hard chair starts hurting my butt after a while. Besides, I start fidgeting in my place thinking I've exceeded my sitting limit and might hurt the baby if I don't go back home and lie down at once. I feel a wetness on the chair and panic, but it turns out it's only my legs sweating in my thick tights and woolen dress in the cozy brasserie and also out of stress... It's lovely to be out and away from the flat (although not so far away) and to have a romantic birthday dinner with my husband, but I can't help it, I can't wait to go home to my white couch. Apparently, I'll have to wait until after delivery to be able to enjoy romantic dinners. I feel safest when I'm home, lying on the couch.*

*During the last month of my pregnancy, we get the doctor's permission to go to the movies. We pick a nice movie. I haven't been to the theater for months and I've missed it so much. But, of course, half way through the movie, I regret my decision to come. I cannot focus on the story because I keep worrying about whether the high volume of sound might affect the baby. I can't help it, I'm ready to give up everything for this baby, even the pleasure of going to the movies, my favorite entertainment! This wasn't a good idea, I think I'd better stick to my couch until term.

My Pregnancy-Related Phobias

Fears and worries fill my pregnant life and surround me wherever I go: fear of catching an infection in the swimming pool; fear of using public restrooms; fear of radiation; fear of moving too much; fear of sitting upright for too long; fear of riding airplanes; fear of exposure to chemicals; fear of lifting heavy objects; fear of food; fear of sonograms, exams, doctors, blood tests and all others lab tests; fear of being in places where they play loud music; fear of trips; fear of all kinds of rides, be it a bike, a train, a bus, or a car... The list goes on... These are the first ones that I can think of.

Normally, I'm a carefree person but pregnancy turned me into a fearful woman. The interesting thing is that what you fear the most in one pregnancy may not bother you in your next one. For instance the Norman Foster Communication Tower case: During my second pregnancy, while I was touring the Tower with my friend Elif (who had paid us a visit in Barcelona on her way back from Valencia where she'd been on an architectural trip), all of a sudden it occurred to me that the radiation in the tower might hurt the baby and I found myself downstairs in a flash. I eventually had a miscarriage but it wasn't because of the radiation, my baby's heart just stopped on the seventh week. When I think of all my meaningless misgivings now, I just smile. But it's simply impossible to overpower your mind at that moment.

During the first trimester of this pregnancy, while I could roam the streets freely, before I'd been confined to stay at home, Cosimo and I went to see a pretty city of Belgium and took a ride on one of those little sightseeing tour trains. I can never forget those fearful minutes. As soon as it began, the bumpy ride on the cobbled street filled my heart with fear and anxiety and I ruined my whole weekend fearing I might have hurt the baby. I knew that the amniotic fluid would protect the baby from such vibrations but I just couldn't help it, I was terrified. The losses I've suffered have left their marks on me, it's so hard to erase them. And you get new phobias once the baby is born, which you eventually get used to as well.

The Gate Is Opened

I can hardly pull my weight around but the cerclage has been removed three days ago and the doctor's given me permission to go out, at long last. So I have to catch up on everything I've been missing during my days at home in just two weeks. I haven't been able to do a thing all throughout my pregnancy, and there are tons of things that I need to do. Although I've been surrounded by my friends willing to help me, there are things that require my own judgment. The baby is soon to come and I'm dying to decorate the nursery for him, but that's going to have to wait. His crib and things are there, and I have to make do with this much for the time being.

My helper, Mrs. Gülten, an experienced mother of three, has washed and ironed all the baby's things and put them away. She's done a good job making the house ready for the baby's arrival. The most urgent thing that needs doing now is for me to prepare my hospital bag, while I still have time. I tell her what I need and she prepares a little suitcase for me. I've read the list of the things that need to go in it in pregnancy books. In the American versions of those books the list is a little too exaggerated to my taste, including playing cards, chess sets, puzzles, stationery to write letters, which I find quite unnecessary. In fact, I am to find out soon that I'm right, you have no time to get bored at the hospital with nurses and staff and visitors coming and going continually in and out of the room.

But I find it useful to take a small notepad, you may want to write down how you feel or to make a list of the things you need. I think I'm already starting to embrace the minimalist way of living that the books encourage you to adopt after the baby's arrival.

✤

Italians believe that the baby's crib and stroller shouldn't be brought in before the baby comes home, lest it bring bad luck. I'm in no hurry, I respect my husband's and his family's superstitions. After all that I've been through, I'm reluctant to rule out bad luck or evil eyes completely myself, you never know. We Turkish have a lot of superstitions, too, we are very similar to Italians in many respects, so I find it natural. We just need the car seat to bring our son home from the hospital, his stroller and crib are in the basement for the time being, where they'll wait until he arrives home. I've really missed being outside, the list of things I want to do starts with walking freely by myself, stopping at a café, and writing while I sip a cup of decaf. It continues with shopping for baby apparel. Of course, almost everything that the baby will need has already been bought by the expectant father, but I want to go around the baby shops and satisfy my motherly instincts.

Since I haven't decorated the nursery, yet, I want to look around to get some ideas. Our flat is very close to the high-street with the classiest shops, which is a great advantage, everything I need is within walking distance. I've missed the social activities of our international women's group during the period I had to spend at home. Although they've often come to see me and never left me alone through my pregnancy, and done everything to help me, I've missed the crowded meetings where you can hear so many languages at once. I've also missed going to the movies with my husband. Although we've done our best to keep abreast of the new award-winning films by watching them at home on DVD's, it's not quite the same as watching them on the big screen.

Life Is Full of Lovely Surprises

It's such a coincidence that my cousin Fethi is in Brussels just on that big day! Our meeting remains in my mind as a great memory. He's in Brussels for a few days on business. As soon as he sees me, "Look at your belly, girl!" he exclaims with his usual silly style of talking, "You are just about to deliver here!"

Cousin Fethi, a cousin from my mother's side and a tour guide, is a very cultured gentleman who graduated from the renowned Galatasaray High school, speaking French as fluently as a native speaker. He'd already been all around the world while he still studied, in those days where you'd find very few people in Turkey who'd ever gone abroad. We used to love to listen to his stories when he stopped by in Tekirdağ once or twice a year. He was charming, and very good looking, turning a lot of heads with those lovely eyes of his. My mother told me that his father, her uncle, may he rest in peace, was very good looking, too. He stole many hearts in Tekirdağ in his day with his striking green eyes. He was a famous tailor in Tekirdağ and an elegant man, starting trends with what he wore. Cousin Fethi, like his father, had a weakness for beautiful women, and one day we heard that he married a celebrated French dancer and moved to Paris, and then to Brussels. Later we heard that he had a son.

One day, after living in Brussels for many years, he decided he just couldn't take it anymore. He was a traveler, of course, and couldn't stay in one place for too long. Brussels didn't satisfy his outgoing Galatasaray spirit and seemed dull to him. He left both Brussels and his French wife and came back to Turkey. When we heard we were to go to Brussels, I called him to talk to as someone who'd spent years there. "So you're appointed to Brussels, of all places!" he said to me with his facetious style, "Bad weather, bad water, a dull place!" That made my day, just before I moved. In time, I saw that he was partly right in what he said. Brussel's erratic weather is unbearable. You wake up to a fine morning, and dress accordingly, but while you're out it starts to rain or a storm breaks out. I've witnessed the weather change in five-minute intervals, it's like a joke. The clouds move in the sky at all speed almost like a time-lapse video, you can go through four different seasons in a day. It's commonplace to be hot then cold, to have sun, and rain, and a storm, and hail during the same day.

The Belgians are used to carrying an umbrella with them, wearing light clothes under their raincoat, and having a scarf or a sweater with them. It would, in fact, make sense if you had a bag of clothes in the car trunk. Yes, Brussels can be dull and boring, even depressive at times. Especially after the shops close after six o'clock in the evening, there is no life anywhere in the city except tourist areas. No one might pass by a street for an hour, if you were attacked and murdered no one would hear or see. You have to go downtown to see more people. But to me, Brussels means so much more. This city has given me both sadness and unparalleled happiness. I cannot be ungrateful to this city where my baby, the love of my life, was born. I've always tried to see it in a favorable light, I've enjoyed all the best it has to give, I've met lovely people, and I've spent four happy years here.

8th March, International Women's Day

I'm at the hospital, my contractions have started. I'm so responsible even in that situation that I cannot believe it myself, still thinking about things that need doing, calls that have to be made, and promises I have to keep! We made an appointment with Paula the midwife to go to a delivery training class, I have to call her and call it off, or it will be awkward... I have to find her phone number somehow. And the most urgent thing to do is to call Cousin Fethi and my neighbor Hülya who I've invited to come over for a glass of wine, and let them know. Where is my cell phone? The nurses tell me to relax and let others think of all that. "Your husband will be here soon," they say. "He'll take care of it all, you just focus on your baby." Easier said than done! I wish I could swap places with one of the nurses and get to give advice to someone just about to give birth! "Excuse me, nurse, have you called my doctor?" I ask – this is just the way I am, I have to take care of all the details before I can take care of myself. "Yes, we have, don't worry," they answer. "Dr. Govaerts will talk to you soon."

It's past eleven o'clock at night. They've put me on epidural, my cervix is opening fast. I finally get to talk to my doctor on the phone: "I'll see you soon, right, you are coming, aren't you?" She answers me of a calm voice: "Don't worry, Nur, you try and get some sleep, so shall I, and I'll see you in the morning," and hangs up. Get some sleep? Seriously? As if I could! She said she'd come in the morning, but what if the baby comes during the night? I think to myself how laid back doctors are! Epidural anesthesia numbs the senses down below the waist but when the contractions come, they really strike, you feel like the baby is coming right away and you panic.

Thank God, they give you a hand held control device that allows you to adjust the dose of the medication to match the intensity of the pain. When I was induced to deliver the twins, the pain made me think that I would give birth at once. I didn't know then, that I might have had to wait for up to 36 hours since the cervix needs to have dilated at least 3.5 inches. But happily four hours later, I was already in the delivery room. I thought delivery was a lengthy process, but mine was over so quickly! I have a hard time conceiving but I think I'm one of those women who deliver easily. This is the one thing my large hips are good for! Because of my previous experience, I have no doubt that I'll deliver easily and quickly this time, too. I'm in good hands and I have to trust them.

The long awaited moment is only a few hours away. The nurses have called my sleeping doctor and started to prep me for delivery. Countdown begins. It's three o'clock in the morning when I'm admitted to the delivery room. There's Dr. Govaerts, in her surgical gown, making preparations. I sigh in relief! She's all awake and alert, with a big smile on her face. "Are we ready?" she asks. Am I ready? Definitely, never been more so. I've been waiting for this moment for days, weeks, months, in fact years on end. I push twice or three times for five minutes or so upon the instructions of my doula and the baby is out at once. I couldn't have even dreamed of such an easy labor. The twins were also born easily but I'd thought it was because they were only 20 weeks old and less than a pound each. I'm surprised a 9 month old baby weighing almost 9 pounds is born so easily. Dr. Govaerts informed me beforehand that she would perform an episiotomy which is an incision on the perineum to facilitate the last stage of labor and to prevent any damage to the perineum muscles. I like the way the

Belgians tell you what they do and why they do it, otherwise how would I know what goes on down there...

Years of waiting, losses, despair, tears, pains, aches, troubles, cuts and sutures, all of that is already fading away into pale memories, it feels like my brain is reset. My heart will beat with a whole new emotion from now on...*

And my baby, my rainbow after the Brussels rain, my sun, my miracle that came at the end of 7 years of waiting, my all, my dearest son, was born at 03.15 a.m. on 9th March.

The Sunrise Has Never Been So Beautiful

Everything was over so quickly! In spite of the long and difficult pregnancy I had to endure, I had a very easy and quick labor and delivery. My son was out of my belly and lying on my chest with his umbilical cord still intact at 03.15 a.m. I was dumbfounded with joy, and I cuddled him clumsily. Astonished, I watched him wriggle on my chest with his warm body, all sticky with amniotic fluid. I witnessed him open his mouth and reach for my breasts with an amazing instinct. They took him away from me for a short while to prepare him for his new world, they cleaned him, took his temperature, checked his heartbeat, weighed and measured him, put on his tiny onesie, hat and booties. They were not done with me yet; they had to take out the placenta, that huge sack the same size as the baby. After checking my womb via sonogram to make it was all clear, there was one last thing to do. As I was on epidural anesthesia, I didn't feel much pain but I could hear the sound of the suture as they stitched the incision. But I was so happy, thinking of my son only, that I didn't care about anything. All I can think of is to have him in my arms again to smell and admire at length. At last, everything was done and we were back in the privacy of our room, with my beautiful son in my arms.

My husband and I watched the sun rise on the morning of March the 9th, with our son lying on my chest. The sun was more beautiful than ever, dying the room a rose color. My son, with his smooth skin and sweet scent, was in my arms. I was thinking to myself that this must be what happiness is. All the moments of happiness I'd had so far were a mere rehearsal for the real thing, an indescribable feeling I was experiencing. I was elated, over the moon. I called my son Matteo, as I had decided months ago, when I read the meaning of the name in Latin, "gift from God." It was the right name for my son, a name that meant much to us. My son was the greatest gift I'd ever received and could ever receive in my life.

He was born with jet black hair that was impossible to guess that would later turn blond. Those who saw my son after a while were not able to recognize him. He was now the one and only prince of our family with his black beads of eyes, vanilla skin and sandy hair.

The morning of my delivery, our first visitors were Cousin Fethi and Hülya who I'd invited over to try some South Italian wine and cheese in our home a day earlier, but we were meant to meet here in a hospital room. They cuddled and held Matteo. I tease Cousin Fethi, saying he caused me to give birth too early with his continuous teasing of my bloated belly, to which he answers, "If I have, it's for the better, now you have your baby in your arms instead of carrying him in your belly." We savor the moment with jokes. My husband is right by me, my son is in my arms. My relatives and friends are there to share my happiness, even though we're in Brussels, twelve hundred miles away from Turkey. I'm only missing my mother, and I have so much to share with her at this moment...*

My Mother

My mother had been expecting her grandson to come 10 days later than he did and she'd planned her visit accordingly. She'd even been thinking she'd arrive a few days early and help with the preparations, when she could actually make it here only two days after he was born. Maybe it was for the best, as I'm sure she couldn't handle the excitement and faint. When I called my parents at night on the 8th of March, I could hear their voice shaking at the other end of the line. They'd thought, like myself, that this moment would never come, but come it had, at long last. It was hard to be miles away and to have to wait for the news. My mother said, "I wish I could be beamed up there at this moment..." Well, she sort of was, if not at that moment just a day later.

---

* In the hours after delivery, when I put my hand on my belly, I found it somehow strange that it was flattened and the baby was out, lying in a crib besides my bed! My son, whom I'd been nursing inside me for 9 months was out of my belly, in my arms. I'd thought I'd never miss being pregnant, but strangely enough, I was already missing my huge belly and being one with my baby. There was a distance of only two feet between my bed and his crib, but the distance would grow with the years to come, and one day he was going to fly away from the nest. I laughed at myself for thinking about this already but I was a mother now; my thinking style had changed, I had jumped into a parallel universe.

The moment she met her grandson was unforgettable. When she took him in her arms she was speechless for a while, then she managed to say, of a shaky voice, and teary eyed, "Oh Lord, I cannot believe it. He's born. My grandson is born." And she admired him quietly for a long while like an art lover admiring an exquisite piece...

My Little Prince is Three Years Old

I cannot believe it! My son who arrived after a long wait of seven years is now three years old as I write this. He is a real blend of Turkish and Italian blood, speaking both languages in a sweet, fluent way. He is a healthy, lively child. Children are beautiful at every age but I think I'd be happy to keep my son at the age of three forever if I could. I never used to understand what my mother meant when she said, "I wish you remained babies and kept to my side." which makes perfect sense to me now. Every age of a child is sweet but when I think he will eventually fly away from the nest I hurt inside and I miss him already.*

* Here is how I put my feelings into words in my column Hola Avrupa in Elele Dergisi Mother's Day Issue of May 2007: My First Mother's Day with my Son...

My quiet pregnancy of 39 weeks is over and my son, whose eyes I was so eager to see, has arrived at long last. We keep looking at one another as if we'd known each other for years... or like lovers who have met after years of separation. Apparently he was eager to see me too, as he came 10 days earlier than expected. My sweet flirt of a son decided he wanted to be born in the midst of a party of 25 lovely women where I was invited on March 8th, International Women's Day. In labor and delivery training classes, when they talk about the signs of the onset of labor, they tell you not to be embarrassed if your water breaks in a public place like a movie theater or a restaurant, as it's only natural. But when it happens to you, it doesn't seem so normal and natural, you panic. The White Couch Disaster! I was sitting on the white couch in the living room of my friend who was throwing the party, engaged in conversation, when my son suddenly decided it was time for him to come out! I flushed crimson instantly, giving away the situation. Those around me, especially keen Esperanza before anyone else, saw my face change color and started screaming of joy: "Are you giving birth?!" I was shedding tears of happiness.

The party which had been moving along calm and peaceful until then suddenly changed pace and everybody was mobilized to rush me to the hospital. When I saw my friends running around in haste in front of the gate, I was seized by a hysterical laugh. I called my husband, who was busy learning Turkish in an evening class in the school of foreign languages. Since I kept laughing on the phone, he didn't believe I was really in labor. My Spanish friend Esperanza was running around like crazy, looking for her car keys, despite the fact that she'd come without her car.... We were all so comical, you had to laugh. Somehow we found another car, on the seat of which I had another gush of water, as if The Disaster of the White Couch was not enough.

And the long awaited guest arrived in five hours, bringing us unparalleled happiness. It's awesome to watch him nurse. Nothing compares to this love, which tops the list of your favorite things at once, and pushing everything else lower, including your husband – no offense. I used to love to enjoy a cup of cappuccino but now my favorite pastime is to watch him suckle at my breast. I never used to miss a party or a new movie but now the time I spend at home with him is much more fun. It's more engaging than any movies to watch his ever-changing facial expressions and his little limbs moving constantly. How shall we spend our Mother's Day? This year, I'll receive greeting calls on Mother's Day. A smile from my son will be the loveliest Mother's Day gift ever. I'll take him for a walk in his stroller as I do every day and watch him drift off to sleep as I push the stroller over the cobbled streets of Brussels, and I'll give thanks for having experienced motherhood, not understanding those mothers who abandon their children...

5

Tekirdağ-Istanbul

March, perhaps by coincidence, has always been a month where great changes happen in my life. My boyfriend proposed in March, I left Istanbul on a snowy day in March, my son was born on a fine day in March. And again, I've received the most surprising news in my life in March. We were having a home party to celebrate Matteo's second birthday, where we'd invited about a dozen of his friends and their parents over. I'd prepared a feast, as I always do every time we throw a party, with separate menus for the kids and the grownups, with any possible party food one can think of... And I couldn't help tasting every dish, just a little bit of this and a little bit of that, I ended up eating a whole lot before the guests had even arrived yet! I couldn't understand what was happening to me those days, I had a voracious appetite!

Soon the guests started showing up with their presents, Matteo was very excited. He ran to the door every time the bell rang. He was too young yet to know what a birthday was, but he could feel that it was a special day. Everybody was there and the children were playing, crawling, and running around like crazy. The gifts were opened, there were wrappers, toys, cookie crumbs all over the place, add to that the screaming kids, and our living room was a battle field. We were prepared to face such a scene so we didn't worry about it too much. The adult guests were also familiar with such scenes, as they were the parents of the little guests, so they took it calmly as well. Matteo and his friends were happy and having a good time, and we parents were having a good time watching them. When the party was over, we were exhausted. The crowd gradually dispersed, and, as I started cleaning up, I took up noshing where I'd left off while I was busy serving and talking to our guests. I felt worn out, which I attributed to the rough day.

❦

My weariness continues in the following days, increasing instead of easing off. And it's the same with my appetite! I can't seem to get satisfied, and after eating I feel so tired that I don't want to lift a finger. I attribute all this to the approaching spring and don't make a big deal out of it. A few days later, a fine sunny morning, my friend Aylin calls to say she's baking a pie and to invite me to come over. She knows I can't say no to pie, but I say I don't feel up to going out and ask her to come over instead, which she does, taking her son Luca with her. I call Patricia too, and she comes with her son Ivan. We're all set. I make tea, I prepare a place for the kids to play in. Cosimo drives to the daycare to pick up Matteo.

Aylin, my skillful cook of a friend, comes with a large platter of hot potato pie that I start drooling over as soon as I see. We set the table, eat pie and drink tea, watching the children in the meantime. What do three boys do when they come together? Either they run around screaming of joy or push each other around. Every now and then we stop to break up a fight over a toy, then we take up our conversation where we'd left off. Being mothers, we've learned to chat in this mess and this noise. My friends are surprised to see the amount of pie I gobble. I tell them I know I eat a lot nowadays, but I can't stop it, I feel hungry all the time, probably because spring is coming. They know I take a spinning class at the gym and work out like crazy, trying to shed the extra pounds I gained during pregnancy. Well, then I shouldn't be eating like this, should I? They start asking me whether I might be pregnant, but I stop them short, saying it's impossible. It's the last thing that could ever happen to me! They must have forgotten how I strived to get pregnant with Matteo!

My eating performance and my energy level follow in this way, until I totally run out of energy. Usually, after I put Matteo to bed around 8.30 in the evening, my night shift starts, I don't sit back but do a lot of work. Both Cosimo and I like staying up late, working, reading and writing in the quiet of the night. But lately I haven't been feeling like myself at all. As soon as I clear the dinner table I quickly retire to my study and curl up like a cat on the cushions in my Ottoman corner, I pull a blanket over me and zap from one Turkish channel to another, alternating between Okan Bayülgen's Sade Vatandaş and Saba Tümer. I call it a day before seeing the end of the shows. I'm not happy spending my precious evening hours in front of the TV screen but I'm so tired and sleepy I don't have the strength to do anything. I tried to wake myself up a few times to no avail.

I wonder if I have some food intolerances like my Italian friend Gian Battista, maybe I'd better have a test done. A few days ago, I was at the swimming pool of the gym I belong to with my Italian friend Stefania, who told me that her husband Gian Battista, who we also call GB, had been waking up tired in the morning, and going through the day with little energy for some time and had decided to see a doctor. The doctor had asked for some tests, which revealed GB was intolerant to wheat and all kinds of cheese, so he was to abstain from these foods for a while and might be able to resume his regular diet when his symptoms vanished. Perhaps it's the same thing with me.

I think of all kinds of explanations but pregnancy. But then I stop and think, could the girls have a point? Could I be pregnant? But I felt I was pregnant straight away in my previous pregnancies, as I was actually trying to conceive and taking hormone supplements to help the process. I've been pregnant four times before, I know very well what you have to do to get pregnant, all the calculations, and all the techniques to increase the odds. But this time, could it be that I got pregnant spontaneously, without any planning, any treatment? No, of course not. That's impossible. That'd be a miracle. On TV, an astrologer says there will be an increase on births and deaths during the early days of March... I tell myself to think positively.

The next morning, after I drive Matteo to daycare, I stop by the pharmacy next door without thinking and get a home pregnancy test kit. I run home to find out the answer to my burning question. Cosimo is home too, since he has been working from home lately as his office is being moved. We love having breakfast together. I'm keeping my cool and not rushing to the bathroom to do the test. We have a full breakfast, taking our time and savoring our delicious lattes that Cosimo has prepared. I tidy up the house, put a load of laundry in the machine, and sit in front of my computer.

Just as I start typing away, my inner voice reminds me of the pregnancy test, I get up, grab the box and run to the bathroom. Oh, how I wish... But I know it's impossible.

I take the test carefully, and the results shows at once. I cannot believe my eyes! The two little parallel bars appear on the tiny window, ever so clear. I didn't expect that! I know what that means but I read the test manual over and over again to be sure, I'm so surprised. I'm pregnant, I cannot believe it! I'm over the moon, I'm definitely one of the happiest expectant mothers at this moment. I never thought this could be possible, but it explains everything, the never-ending fatigue, my hearty appetite, my breasts becoming fuller and tender... So, you can get pregnant this easily! This pregnancy that I haven't planned or expected in the least, which comes all by itself, for free, if I may say so, without any struggle on my part, is the greatest surprise of my life. I run at once to break the news to my husband, who's engrossed in the world market news he's viewing on his computer screen. When he sees my beaming face, he looks at me with anticipation and asks me what it is. I tell him I'm pregnant. He didn't expect that! His eyes gleam with joy, he gives me a passionate hug and kiss. We stand staring at each other for a while.

"I still can't believe it," I say, "how did this happen!" My darling husband replies, "So it can happen. Apparently we are both free from stress these days, with me working at home instead of going to the bank, and leading a peaceful, stress-free life with my family, and you having relaxed because you already have a baby." We strived and struggled, put up with so much, went through so much pain and trouble for seven years... seven! And one day I find myself pregnant just like that. I still can't believe it. So, it's just that easy to get pregnant, no doctor's appointments, no counting days, no drugs, no ovulation monitoring, no lying on exam chairs. How easy, how nice it is to get in bed just to make love, and to make a baby without thinking about the day or the time, without worrying about ovulation, just like that! So, what are we going to do now? The situation is a little tricky, we've heard about Cosimo's appointment to Italy only days ago and have to move to Italy in a few months. So much news in such a short time.

I have to see my doctor at once. I must still be at the very beginning of my pregnancy but I'd like to make sure everything is going well. Perhaps I have to start taking folic acid, hormone supplements and vitamins right away. Have done anything that could hurt the baby these days? Have I, for instance, had too many glasses of wine? Have I fallen ill and taken any medicine? I'd been planning ahead to get pregnant for years before, taking folic acid for months on end, but now I've been happy raising my little boy, completely free from care, and definitely not planning to have another baby, so folic acid is not a part of my life anymore. I must admit, I had doubts about having a second baby, as I had so many difficulties to have my first one. But it got me by surprise. I explain the situation to my doctor's assistant and secure an appointment in three days, which is quite a short time with respect to Belgian standards. I'm used to waiting. I've waited so many hours in years for my turn to come in hospitals, doctors' offices, health care centers, laboratories... patiently, anxiously, and always hopefully, wishing to have a baby...

The longest three days of my life... We are in the hospital with Cosimo to see our doctor and meet our baby. I know it's too early yet and the baby is so small I can't possibly see anything, but I'm still willing to wait for hours to see that black dot of a baby on the sonogram. Dr. Isabelle Govaerts, my pretty and cool ob-gyn, meets us at the door of her office, with her usual big smile, and lets us in saying, "Congratulations, what great news! I'm so happy for you." I still can't believe it, I think it's a miracle, whereas she finds it quite natural. "There are so many women in your situation," she says, without blinking, "so many miracles. We see such pregnancies all the time." I was on infertility treatment just about two years ago, but now it's the other way around: if I can get pregnant that easily I may have to use contraceptives! "It's very common," she says! Well, it isn't, it is extraordinary! I too have heard many stories but I've never suspected it could happen to me. Dr. Govaerts says, "You see, Nur, haven't I always told you to make another baby without waiting too long. This time nature has helped you, it gave you chance without waiting for you to make plans. It's for the best, believe me when I say that a woman your age shouldn't lose time if she wants another baby, time is not on your side."" I tell her that we didn't expect this at all and it got us totally by surprise.

I remind her that I had to spend my previous pregnancy in bed and ask her what I will need to do this time. She replies that it's not necessary that I stay in bed but advises me to lie down and rest as much as can. "But I have a two year old son," I say, "how's that going to be?" She tells me to think of the baby I'm carrying for the time being and everything else will sort itself out. I want to believe her, but I can't help feeling overwhelmed. I'm pregnant, and we have to move in a few months' time. Matteo clings to me, he's always on my lap or right next to me; I can't lose him even in the house, we live stuck together. He's a little lamb, he's too young yet, he's not old enough to cope by himself. He wants attention and needs care. So how am I supposed to lie down and rest? Easier said than done! When I tell her all this, Dr. Govaerts says, "Your husband, your family will have to support you. Everybody will make a little sacrifice, and your little son will understand that he will be a big brother soon." And then she adds, "You will be under less stress about your pregnancy this time as you already have a child. But you'll have to take good care of yourself nevertheless. Don't you carry things around while you are moving house, let your husband do the work, you are carrying a baby and that's as much load as you can handle."

I ask her what I need to be doing at this stage. It's like I'm pregnant for the first time, I've forgotten all about it, it's all new to me... In fact, this is what makes it so nice... My doctor explains: "We'll do the same thing as we did when you were pregnant with Matteo. The precautionary measures we took then worked fine and you've had a healthy pregnancy and a healthy baby. It's a must that we give you a cervical cerclage around the 12th to the 14th week. We don't need to do amniocentesis as you are under 40, we usually don't do that test to women under 40 in Belgium." Yes, but we're just about to move from Belgium to Treviso in Italy, where Cosimo has to start in his new position in a month. A new home, a new life, a new job, new friends, a brand new start to everything...

Cosimo, well organized as he is, comes up with an alternative plan at once. He is going to find our new house in Italy and deal with the moving. I cannot really do much in this turmoil with my bulging belly and my baby son. Besides, the most important thing right now is the health of the baby growing in my belly, moving will be done somehow. Therefore the best thing to do seemed for me to go and stay with my family in Turkey until delivery. It's popular among the wealthier in Turkey to go abroad, especially to the USA, to give birth, and here I am going back to Istanbul to give birth instead of Italy or Belgium. Well, I wouldn't know about the other Turkish cities but I have total confidence that I'll be very well looked after in Tekirdağ or Istanbul. I have visited the obstetrics ward of the Public Hospital in Tekirdağ and I was convinced that we are good at this delivery business in Turkey, well, we are a country with a very high fertility rate after all, and to think a million and a half babies are born in Turkey every year! We'll run circles around any other country in population growth!

The unutterable happiness Matteo brought into our life was more than enough for me. My maternal instincts were completely satisfied. In truth, I didn't plan on having a second baby. I'd struggled so much to have a baby that I felt too tired to start all over again. My pregnancy had been very difficult, it was scary to think of another pregnancy that I would have to spend in bed. Matteo took up a good part of my time. My husband always said he liked large families but he never put any pressure on me about it. If I ever thought of having another baby, I guess it would be for the sake of my husband and my son but it was too early to think about it yet. Besides, it was totally a bad time to attempt to have another baby as we were on the verge of moving to a different country. Even if we decided to engage in fertility treatment, it was a lengthy process, and a serious one. For all these reasons, I didn't feel like trying to have a baby and I didn't feel up to it. I kept telling myself I'd think of it when the right time came... The news that I was pregnant came just then, sorting everything out at once and completing

the family picture. The second baby had entered our life on his own,
there was no need to give it much thought, no dilemma to fret about.
The 'bonus' baby had selected me as its mother. I was so lucky.

A Ten-Minute Operation

As Dr. Yücel Karaman has a full schedule, my cervical cerclage
surgery has been arranged to take place at noon. He comes to
Brussels for only a few days a month due to the number of his
patients in Istanbul, yet manages to handle so much in such a
limited time, including my 10-minute operation, he's a hero. He's
definitely not one of those materialistic doctors who start to care
less about their patients as they grow popular. On the morning of
the surgery, I'm first admitted to my room and prepped for surgery.
This time I will only be locally anaesthetized with epidural instead
of full anesthesia, therefore I don't need to be give an enema, of
which I keep terrible memories. An attendant had me lie down on
a gurney and wheeled me past the corridor, into an elevator, past
another corridor, into another elevator, and finally to the operation
room in a lower floor of the building.

Rows of patients, lying on gurneys, prepped for surgery, are
waiting in the cold, white reception area with a high ceiling, outside
of the operation room. We constituted a grotesque, unreal scene,
lying on gurneys, half naked in hospital gowns, waiting to have an
operation, like lambs for slaughter. You know when they use an ice-
blue filter in sci-fi movies to create a cold, creepy effect, that's was
the atmosphere. Everyone is taken in the operation room when
their turn comes and the row of gurneys keep moving forward.
When it's my turn, the nurse who comes to take me in wants to

confirm that I haven't had anything to eat in the morning... but I have! How stupid of me to have thought it was alright to have breakfast as the operation was scheduled to be around noon. But it turns out you have to wait for at least five hours so you can digest what you've eaten. So I'm sent to the end of the line. I have to lie there and watch all the other patients to be taken in for surgery, to come out, and new patients to come around.

In the meantime, Dr. Govaerts and Dr. Karaman keep getting in and out of the surgery room every thirty minutes or so. Once they notice me and ask after me, and I tell them I have to wait because I've had breakfast. My witty doctor teases me, asking what I had for breakfast, which question I take seriously and dutifully answer: "Feta cheese, bread, and decaf coffee." I'm so nervous that my doctor continues his teasing: "You've had feta cheese! Turkish feta, too?" Guilty and gullible to the fullest, I reply earnestly. This test and that, this surgery and that, local or full or epidural anesthesia, do this, do that, sutures to be put in, sutures to be removed, come with an empty stomach, come full, have plenty to drink, load up on sugar... I all confused! I've had just a little something to eat, and I regret it bitterly! I congratulate myself to manage to lie there on that gurney in that cold room, without getting up once and without losing patience, for six hours on end, at the end of which I'm admitted to the operation room and it's all over in 15 minutes. So, that was it, I forgot all about my first time around. Dr. Karaman sutures my cervix with his magical hands. For the attention of my baby: Baby dearest, I'm closed until your arrival. You are safe in there, so don't you worry!

Group for Mothers

In Brussels, we had a lovely group of Turkish mothers, which we had started with Binnur, whom I'd met in a labor training class organized by the hospital. My due date was the 16th of March and hers the 9th, but our actual delivery dates turned out just the other way around. We had a lot in common, we were both seeing the same doctor, we were both Turkish, we both had international marriages, both of us had moved to Brussels because of our husbands' jobs and decided to realize our dream of having a baby here in Brussels; all of which brought us closer. As two expectant mothers, our favorite topic of conversation was labor and delivery and nothing else!

Once, Binnur told me about a mothers society established by British women and invited me to an event where mothers and babies were meeting to socialize. I couldn't say our British host treated us too hospitably, which made us decide to establish our own Turkish mothers group. An added benefit would be for the little ones to be exposed to and get to practice their mother tongue more often, while they played together. Binnur had told me about Aylin whom she'd met over the Internet, and who happened to be one of my first friends in Brussels. Everyone let the other Turkish friends of theirs with babies know of the meetings, so the "Turkish Mothers in Brussels" group was formed almost on its own. The group members mixed and mingled easily, we organized morning events and afternoon teas, the kids played and capered, the mothers conversed and exchanged information; we appeased our longing for our own culture and language.

Every time I was pregnant, I kept it a secret for the first trimester lest I'd miscarry. Aylin, being very close to me, figured it out, even before I knew it myself, seeing me devour the pie she'd made. I would like to share the good news with all the group, but every time I started to tell I drew back. What was stopping me was not only the fact that I wasn't through the first trimester yet; I was also afraid to cause pain to our friend Gonca, who had a problem. She was pregnant with her second baby but the doctors suspected that it wasn't growing healthily. Gonca was having a rough period, troubled with anxiety and fear of losing the baby and we were trying to be supportive, meeting often to cheer her up. I could understand exactly how she felt as I'd been through it myself in the past. She was going to move to Geneva soon due to her husband's new assignment, so we met in a pizzeria for a goodbye dinner. No one noticed me order a non-alcoholic beer to drink. I was dying to tell everyone I was pregnant, but I couldn't. We were all a little sad that night, both because we had to say goodbye to Gonca, and because we were all worried about the five-month old baby that she carried. We were all teary eyed, it was not a good time to share happy news. I couldn't be so selfish as to expect anyone to share my happiness while we had to share someone else's sadness...

Matteo is Learning To Love His Unborn Sibling

Matteo is watching in surprise as my belly grows larger from day to day, and understands that he will soon have a baby brother or sister. When I tell him he's going to be a big brother soon, he smiles, opens his arms, and says, "Baby!" When he wants to nurse I tell him his brother will need my breasts when he comes, and he tries to express that he wants to feed his brother by saying, "Baby, breast, food." I'm already giving him little tasks to do to get him involved, like rubbing cream on my belly, bringing me drinks of water or fruit juice, and giving me a back rub with his tiny hands when I complain about a backache. He sometimes even lays me down on the couch and tries to lull me to sleep. Apparently, he is taking over his father's tasks this time around. He's taking great care of me during my pregnancy. I'm trying to familiarize him with the idea that he will have a brother or sister, who will be a great friend to him.

I want to prevent him from getting traumatized when his brother arrives. I know it's unavoidable that he will feel jealous, as the arrival of a new baby while he's still this young and in need of care and attention will end his absolute reign in the house, dividing my life, my time, my attention and my energy into two. Perhaps we will not be able to do the things he wants to do at once, like we do now. He will be jealous because he will experience the fear of losing his mother to someone else, maybe he will try to hurt the baby, probably subconsciously, to get my attention. He will think, in revolt, 'Where did this baby come from, stealing mommy away!' Perhaps he'll think his mother doesn't love him anymore, he'll want to nurse too while I nurse the baby, he'll want to sit on my lap while I hold his brother, he'll show irritable, aggressive and angry behavior. He'll think the baby is taking his place. I can foresee all this and I'm well prepared!

But for the time being, my sweet, smart boy is excited, looking forward to his baby brother's arrival, I know that. He tiptoes to me in the morning, saying "Hush, the baby is asleep." When he wants to tumble with me on the big bed, he knows I'll warn him to be careful about the baby, so he says it before me: "Careful with the baby, mom." Although he's showing his love for the baby and his desire to be a big brother, I can still foresee what will happen. The experts say that jealousy usually starts at the age of two and onwards, and increases after the age of four or five. Your child needs more love and attention during this period, and you have to express your love verbally as well as showing it. Matteo is my first born, my dear son! How could I do less than showing and telling him that I love him all the time!

Last Days in Brussels...

I love travelling but I hate packing up! It's as stressful to try to compact your wardrobe into a suitcase, especially when you have to do it with two kids, as it's exciting to be going somewhere. It's going to be even harder to pack up to go to Turkey, as I have to pack three seasons of clothing for my son and me both, and in different sizes! How am I supposed to do that! We are going to have to go through summer, fall and winter until delivery, and I have to have a maternity wardrobe to suit my ever-changing size and shape. I start with paying a visit to H&M's maternity department. Then I open the famous green chest Cosimo bought from an antiques shop in Moscow, where I've been keeping Matteo's clothes that he grew out of, not knowing when they might come in handy... Well, that time has come quicker than I expected. I'm through the 14th week of my pregnancy and I don't know the baby's gender yet.* If it's a boy, he won't need a thing, if it's a girl, it's all the same, as the newborn clothes are mostly white in color. We put everything we'll need for the first month in the suitcase.

A Farewell Dinner of Mussels & French Fries...

I'm about to leave Belgium, where I've spent my last four years, my heart is heavy with sentiment. I've shed a lot of tears in this city, but I've also had my son here, who is the meaning of my life. Belgium is a small country but filled with immigrants from all over the world, so there is a large international community. There is no denying that there is some degree of racism here too, like any other European country. As foreigners living in Europe, we've come to accept it as a fact. But I could hear many people talking in Turkish in the streets in Brussels, as there is quite a large Turkish community, and it was a great comfort to me, I didn't feel alone. When I felt homesick, I could always go to the Turkish quarter** and appease my longing, eating a simit† with a drink of ayran.‡

*** Years ago, when Belgium needed Turkish workers to work in the mines, many Turkish families immigrated here, and not many went back. They had children and grandchildren, some of them even*

---

* The results of the double and triple tests I have done during the last days of our stay in Brussels reveal that it's a boy. We are so happy, it's going to be a best friend for our Matteo. He will wear his big brother's clothes, the garments I've put in the suitcase will come to good use.

† A Turkish bread, in the shape of a ring, covered with sesame seeds.

‡ A savory drink of yoghurt diluted with water.

called their relatives to come and join them in Belgium, when their children got married in Turkey, they had their sons- and daughters-in-law come to live with them. All the Turkish people I come across in Brussels turn out to be from Emirdağ, a district of Afyon province. You would think the citizens of Emirdağ moved to Brussels all together. I'd never met someone from Emirdağ during the 35 years I spent in Turkey, while I met so many of them in Brussels. Immigrants usually lead a closed, introverted life in their new countries, without completely adapting to the life there. Especially women who do not work but stay at home will spend their whole life without learning a single word of the country's language, how they do it is a mystery I cannot understand. They say there are about 300,000 Turkish people living here, but they live in their own quarters and communities, without mingling much with the Belgians.

We are in Le Pré-Salé for a farewell dinner. This is a place we discovered the first night of our Christmas holiday in Brussels, a butcher's shop turned into a mussel restaurant that struck our eye while we were wandering in the streets. They served 'Moules & Frites', a traditional Belgian dish consisting of a casserole of mussels with crispy French fries. I like to try the local cuisine in the places I visit and Moules & Frites was on my list for that trip. When we walked into the crowded restaurant, I saw people fishing mussels with their hands from inside large pans, but it didn't turn me off, it even whetted my appetite. As we lived in Barcelona then, we were accustomed to having our dinner late at night, and we were happy to see that some customers who'd had their dinner early were already leaving so we could be seated.

We were surprised to learn that the restaurant opened at 18.30 and wondered who would want to eat that early in the evening. (But here we are tonight, among those early diners, as we are now a family with child.) We took our table just by the door and at a distance of a few inches with the next table, without complaining. We laughed, thinking of the reactions that such a sitting arrangement might attract in Turkey or Italy. Nevertheless, the food was exquisite. I had Moules à la Provençale (mussels stewed with vegetables such as tomatoes, carrots and celery stalks, deliciously juicy) and Cosimo had mussels cooked in white wine, both dishes served with a side of golden crisp French fries and ice cold Belgian beer Vedett.

After we have moved to Brussels, we've tried all kinds of restaurants and dishes, in the pursuit of local tastes. We asked the locals, when we particularly liked a restaurant we met the owners, we asked for their personal addresses, we tasted their special dishes and took the recipes. The Europeans are free from cunning, they are at peace with themselves. The owner of a restaurant might recommend another one without worrying about losing customers, because he knows his cuisine is good, he's confident that his customers will come back.

This time we are in Le Pré-Salé for a farewell dinner as a family of four, including Matteo and the baby in my belly. Cosimo has Moules & Frites and beer, while I, abstaining from mussels because of my pregnancy, order sole in butter sauce and French fries, and chicon (Belgian endive) salad that I love, even though the Turkish in Belgium are not very keen on it. It's a pleasure to watch my two year old son sit on chair and eat from his own plate like a grownup in a restaurant. In Belgium, all restaurants have a children's menu. Matteo ate up his menu of fried fish fillet and mashed potatoes successfully by himself, with very little help. We are saying farewell to Brussels with a real feast that we enjoy both with our palates and with our eyes. Brussels, the city of Matteo and his brother! Goodbye for now, even though we don't like to say farewell!

Passengers for Turkey, All Aboard!

Our last days in Brussels... One morning, Cosimo finds he cannot get up from bed, it's his herniated disc that troubles him now and then. Tough luck, just when I needed him! How is he going to take care of us when he can't take care of himself? It takes just one phone call to my mother for her to jump on the plane and come to our rescue. Dearest mother, she's known for her unhurried way, but she can act like a blue streak when it comes to her daughter!

Travelling with a child brings an extra burden, especially when you are pregnant, and you have nothing to do but take it lightly or you'll go crazy. We leave our house in Brussels to go to Istanbul on the morning of May 31st, with six suitcases. Jean-Pierre, our landlord, who has risen early in the morning to see us go, is helping load the luggage in the cab. We are all subdued. We've known we were leaving Brussels, our home, our landlord for a long time but you can never be ready for the moment of departure. Both I and Jean Pierre are tearful, we hug each other and start to cry. We jump into the cab hurriedly, so as not to prolong this scene. I knew it was unavoidable, how could I leave our home filled with memories bitter and sweet, and the city where I lost the twins and gained Matteo, without shedding tears! My mother is used to seeing me cry but she's astonished to see our landlord join me, she says "Jean Pierre is literally crying," in amazement while she keeps waving at him until the cab rounds the corner of the street.

We make it to the airport easily. But, good Lord! A line stretches away in front of the check-in desk to an invisible distance. I couldn't possibly wait in this line when I shrink from standing longer than five minutes at a time and slouch in the nearest chair; I'd probably deliver on the spot! The only solution I can think of is to go the Turkish Airlines office and tell them about my situation. They are very sympathetic and they take me in through the business-class check-in desk. There is no reason why I shouldn't make use of the advantages pregnancy brings, but I can tell the other passengers in the queue resent the special treatment I receive, as my belly doesn't really show yet. I can see they cannot understand why I shouldn't have to wait, but it's the health of the baby that matters most, I don't care about the rest. This is how I have been feeling lately, totally careless about anything else than my baby boy and the baby in my belly.

We go to passport control after check-in, fortunately I'm able to go through the disabled gate thanks to Matteo's stroller. Before we can sigh in relief, we have to go through the security check next, and the line is at least three or four times as long as the check-in line. Once more, I explain my special situation to the attendants, who tell me they can let me go in front of the line, but my mother and son will have to wait. I don't have a choice, but to say yes to the woman attendant with a very brusque stance, talking in a curt manner. Thankfully, they give me a chair to sit down on, but I still feel I've been standing too long and drown in anxiety.

I see my mother and Matteo come through the security gate after waiting for almost 45 minutes. My mother has a long face,

Matteo is bored to death. We have to proceed to the gate at once, or we will miss the plane. Fortunately, since all passengers are late, the takeoff is delayed. My son has a seat of his own between ours since he's over the age of two, he puts on his seat belt with dexterity. Children are very smart nowadays. And it's a relief for me to travel without a child on my lap, I can even have hot coffee and read! Although it doesn't come for free, you have to pay a fee comparable to that of an adult ticket for a child over the age of two.

Then, just as I sit back and relax, I feel something drip on my hair. Oh my God! It's the sweat from the brow of the man who's trying to put his bag in the overhead compartment just above me! I run to the lavatory, heaving in disgust. No wonder my mother prefers a window seat, now I learned my lesson... I come back to find a naughty boy sitting in front of us provoking my well-behaved son, waving his toy gun and sword in his face and going, "boom!" We are about to take off, his mother and the flight attendants try to make the boy who wants to play war sit down, to no avail. The situation looks pretty hopeless, the mother has a nervous breakdown and starts yelling at her son, but thankfully he finally calms down. A good number of the passengers on our flight are elderly Turkish workers living in Belgium with their families, they are dressed in too many layers despite the weather, and some faint as their blood pressure goes up due to the heat.

The man whose sweat dripped on my head is now watering his mother's head with it. We giggle with my mother. The man's mother is feeling faint because of the heat and all the layers of clothing she's wearing. Turkish Airlines has thought of everything for children, they give a gift pack of toys to all children as they board the plane, which entertains the kids for almost an hour. Then they serve refreshments, which distract them for a while, then they play with the toys they've brought with them, and the two hour flight is over without trouble. We're finally drifting down over Istanbul. Flights usually don't bother me but flying when I'm pregnant is different, more worrying. I kiss and nuzzle my baby son sleeping with his head on my lap, it's like his warm presence braces me. My mother smiles sweetly as if to comfort me. I sigh in relief as we finally land and our adventurous journey ends without any major mishaps. My father and brother are waiting for us in the airport, and we hold each other lovingly.

Tekirdağ Diary

I can't wait to sink in the swing in the garden of our summer house in Tekirdağ after leaving our house in Brussels and having an adventurous flight with my mother and son, and our six suitcases and two strollers. Despite all my efforts to calm myself throughout the journey, I can't help feeling anxious. You can think of weird things when you are pregnant, you can invent such scenarios as could make great thrillers or horror movies. I fear that my membranes might rupture, that the vibrations in the plane might travel through the amniotic fluid and hurt the baby. What if we encounter air turbulence? If the plane shakes violently, would it shake the baby in my belly? Would the drop of pressure affect the baby as the plane rises? Have I been on my feet too long in the airport? Have I walked too much? I know I'm just obsessing, but I can't help it. I've looked it up, read about it, asked the doctor, even read about it in the newspaper in the plane, I know flying doesn't hurt the baby in the womb, but tell this to my brain!

It's as if we were moving to the summer house in Tekirdağ for good, even though we are here to stay only for a short period. I know I can find everything in Turkey, but I still carry around many things I got used to in Brussels. I'm a Cancer by sign, I move around with my shell like a crab, carrying my home around wherever I go and making any place I go into a home. And, of course, I'm Turkish. I'm not very good at giving up my habits and want everything to be in immediate reach. So I have with me my son's Belgian diaper rash cream, his nail clippers, and the pink vitamin pills I'll be using through pregnancy, my hair brush, everything from soup to nuts! And that's after eliminating most items that were previously on the list, no less! I hope we can go through our stay of six months with six giant suitcases...

When you have a child, you have to establish a child-friendly setting wherever you go. His bed time, his bath time, his meal times, his play time... as a mother, you have to see to all that, and more. We used to come here every summer, and we didn't really need to bring much with us, as we only came to stay for a short while. But we are staying longer this time, at least seven months, so we have to have a permanent setting. We get a new bed for Matteo's room, a new dresser for the extra clothes, a second air-conditioner, an inflatable kiddy pool for the courtyard, and a comfortable lounger for me, and we're alright for the time being. Of course, we also need to have a tap installed in the courtyard to fill the kiddy pool. The sun filtering through the blinds and waking me up early in the morning gets on my nerves, as I'm already having a hard time sleeping at night because I'm having trouble regulating my body temperature due to hormonal imbalances, getting hot and cold alternately, so we have the window fitted with curtain rods and thick curtains. The night lamp is not bright enough for me to read, so we get a new night light.

Even though the room is air-conditioned, you have to open the window to let fresh air in, doing which you also let mosquitoes in! And they are very partial to my blood, they seem to come directly to me to sting even in a crowded room. That's another job for you, we have to have the windows fitted with mosquito screens. The house teems with plumbers, air-conditioner installers, furniture delivery people, carpenters, curtain fitters, and electricians. We've totally turned the house upside down. My saintly parents shrink from no sacrifice for the sake of their daughter and grandson. We are finally settled at the end of the second week.

It's June and the days are nice and warm, and Matteo and I enjoy the beach and the sea. His favorite pastime is playing with our dog Çakır, collecting snails from the garden and proudly giving them to me. He also likes to pluck the lovely hydrangeas that my father grows with love and care and brings them to his mother, the fine gentleman that he is. He fills his little bucket with whatever he finds on the sand, then he empties it, and starts over times on end, without ever getting bored. He wants to go on the little boats moored at the shore and play captain. I love the way he salutes like a captain with his little hands. He likes to join his granddad on his rounds to the farm, where he can see and pet the farm animals, and feed them of his own hands. He loves picking plums from the orchard, he gives them out to us, calling our names one by one. He spends the whole day in his swimming suit, so he can dig into a slice of watermelon with the juices running down his wrists and elbows, free from care.

His hair is curly, with sweet locks, and everybody loves it even more as it grows longer. Some even mistake him for a girl. We decide for him to get a haircut and take him to his uncle's classy barber. His uncle goes through the door of the barber shop proudly with his nephew on his shoulders. But the pride vanishes as soon as Matteo sits on the barber chair and starts to cry inconsolably, not wanting to have his hair cut. We swallow the failure and head back, to try some other day.

Despite so much activity and fun, the pleasures of the sea and the beach, the attention of his grandparents, I realize that, after a while, my son starts missing the company of friends of his own age, but there aren't any other kids of his age around the neighborhood. Matteo started daycare when he was a year and a half and he is used to being among his peers, so I decide to put him in a playschool here. I visit a few summer schools and find a good one for him. He fits in quickly despite the unfamiliar surroundings, and he becomes the favorite of the teacher and the trainees as he always does, sociable and friendly as he is.

He wakes up early in the morning and runs straight to my bedside. He wakes me up with a kiss and says "Good morning!" He is so convincing with his sweet smile that I oblige, getting up even if I'm dying to sleep a little more. My thoughtful son puts my slippers on my feet, and we go down to the living room to play. The fact that children wake up with a desire to play first thing in the morning always amazes me. Oh, the things you will do for your child, one of which is playing games even in the small hours of the morning! Then we prepare a big breakfast, which we have on the terrace with a full view of the beach, and then I see Matteo off to playschool with his granddad. The time he spends at the playschool is my 'me-time', where I do my writing and relax. If it's a sunny day, I bask in the sun in the garden or go for a walk on the beach. The salty sea water is good for circulation. As I'm not allowed to do any heavy exercise, I like to walk in the sea for a while, which is good workout for the legs and muscles. After moderate workout, it's time to take to a corner with my laptop and write for at least a few hours. In the afternoon, my dearest son comes home and wants to play with his mother with his never-ending energy. As the evening wears on, I start to run low on energy, but I work hard to fulfill my son's wishes. After all, it's a critical period for him, he's going to have a brother, and he shouldn't feel neglected and be jealous.

I'm along the fourth month of my pregnancy and my morning sickness is finally over. How horrible it is to have to live with a heaving stomach all the time. You don't enjoy anything you eat or drink, it makes it hard even to go to bed and sleep. I try to have my dinners early in the evening throughout my pregnancy. Although morning sickness subdues after the first trimester, stomach problems continue throughout pregnancy. The uterus growing larger as the baby grows puts pressure on the stomach, which, coupled with the relaxation of the valve that separates the esophagus from the stomach owing to pregnancy hormones, causes heartburn, or acid reflux. Oh, those hormones! To keep my stomach comfortable and prevent it from spoiling my sleep, I try to avoid large meals and eat several light meals, and, most importantly, I try and have my dinner early. Not that I never slip, sometimes I do eat late at night or have a whole large slice of watermelon just before I go to bed, sometimes guiltily, sometimes recklessly... But I pay dearly

for it every time, as I toss and turn in bed, unable to sleep because of
heartburn. Thank God I have to deal with this only at night and only
during pregnancy. There are some who suffer from it their whole life!
How hard it must be!

"So, It's Another Boy?" "Well, Nevermind..."

I wonder what gender the babies I lost were. I know that of the
twins, one was a boy and the other one a girl. I have Matteo and
another son to be born soon. So I know the genders of four babies,
one girl and three boys, but I wonder what the other four were.
If they could have been born, what would they look like? Perhaps
some were blond, with green eyes, with both their grandmothers,
some with jet black hair and brown eyes like myself. And what
would they be like, logical, calm and patient like their father or
creative, impulsive and outgoing like their mother?

In our grandparents' generation, boys were more valued than
girls, they were considered important for the continuation of the
family name. My parents' generation was the first to value girls too,
whereas in our generation girls are definitely more popular, even
though I see boys all around. I guess one of the factors fuelling the
popularity of girls is the baby clothing industry; when you see the
most fashionable items in tiny sizes in the shop windows, you just
want to go and buy them, whether you have a baby girl or not. I
(and other mothers of boys like me) used to go to DOD, Brussels
best baby clothing magazine, and buy sweet baby girls' garments
to give to friends who had daughters.

I'll have another son. I'm elated about it, but, I see others
don't consider it good news, their comments make me smile. The

dialogue usually goes as follows: "Have you found out the baby's gender yet?" I answer, "Yes, Matteo is going to have a baby brother." And they go, "Oh, I wish it was a girl... Well, olsun..." And then silence. That olsun makes me laugh to myself, I have a hard time to translate it into Italian for my husband. It's such a Turkish idiom, so versatile and so humble, the direct translation would be "let it be," but the feeling it expresses is accepting a mediocre outcome without complaining, or making the best of a bad thing, more like "never mind," like a consolation in the face of something that cannot be changed. What I'm finding hard to understand is what those who 'olsun' me want to console me for.

As a woman who struggled for years to have a baby, this 'bonus baby,' as my doctor calls it, is such a lovely surprise, the best thing that could ever happen to me. Who cares about the gender! I find it absurd to even talk about it. This second baby has come as a surprise to both of us as a couple, but if I had planned to have another baby at all, it would have been to give a sibling to my son, so he wouldn't grow up as an only child, not for myself, because I'd already satisfied my desire to be a mother. Now we are having a second baby and it's a boy, could life get any better? A brother, a playmate. Besides, it's an economic boon for the family, you can easily raise your second son with the hand-me-down clothes, toys, and belongings of the first one, without spending an extra penny. The comments from those who hear it's going to be another boy are usually along the lines of "too bad it's not a girl," but fortunately there are some who find it nice that I'll have another son and who agree with me that it's a good thing. When I tell Cenk, my childhood friend and colleague, that I'm expecting a baby boy again, he says, "Oh, great news! He's going to be a good friend to Matteo," because he has a brother, 3 years younger, and they had a great, fun childhood together and they have always been best friends.

My Pregnancy with Three Doctors

The first thing I did when I arrived in Tekirdağ was to find myself a doctor. I'd had a trouble-free pregnancy and felt safe all through the last time thanks to my cautious doctor in Brussels. Although I was planning to go to Istanbul for delivery, I had to have a doctor in the city where I lived. Dr. Govaerts, my doctor in Brussels, felt the same way. The last time I saw her, she recommended for me to find a doctor in Tekirdağ immediately as I arrived, to oversee my pregnancy. Dr. Levent was a young and successful doctor renowned in Tekirdağ.

My father accompanied me to my first appointment. He was just as excited as I was. The doctor's assistant welcomed us cordially and let us in the reception area, decorated and furnished like a living room, with a view of the sea, where we sank in the comfortable chairs. We only had to wait about five minutes, the appointments were very well organized. The doctor's assistant saw the patient before us off and then led us into the doctor's office. The patient after us who arrived just before we were out was let into the reception area to wait a few minutes, and this went on like that smoothly and peacefully, without anyone having to wait too long or too many patients crowding the reception area. I was fed up with waiting endlessly for doctor's appointments in hospital and clinic reception areas for years, I wasn't used to such smooth operation, it felt great. The doctor was young and energetic and kind, and he had an energy, a voice and a smile that instilled confidence and peace in you. After a few cordial words of introduction, he said he was ready to listen to my medical history.

I tell my long and complicated story all over again, in full detail, like I do with every new doctor. As I have committed all the figures to memory I just tell them flawlessly without even thinking: one cervical infection surgery, five pregnancies in total, two deliveries with epidural anesthesia, two cervical cerclage operations, one corrective surgery of the uterus, and six babies lost in between... But there are also the nice figures, I have a 27 month old, healthy, good-looking son, and I'm four months pregnant with a second son. I had a miscarriage in Istanbul, two deliveries in Barcelona, this hospital and that, it's hard even for me to remember, naturally enough, the doctor is a little confused with all these complicated details so he has to ask me to repeat some points. I shouldn't think he has any other patients with such a medical history within Tekirdağ.

We do an ultrasound and while I'm busy admiring the baby floating with soft motions in the sack, my father is curiously examining the numbers on the screen. The doctor carefully takes the necessary measurements and says everything looks fine and healthy. The level of amniotic fluid is fine, and there's an adequate distance between the baby's head and the cervix. I sigh in relief. These are the two issues that worry me most; the level of amniotic fluid and the distance between the baby's head and the cervix... My father is not familiar with sonograms as they didn't have them in my mother's time, he asks the doctor if there is any health risks for the baby. The doctor explains that it involves only sound waves reflected from various parts of the baby and put together with the ultrasound machine to form a monochromatic image and that it doesn't harm the baby or the mother in any way. He gives my father picture of the 18 week old 'Submarine 2,' my father looks at it with a beaming face, unable to put it down.

The doctor presents me with his card, with his hospital, office and private numbers, telling me I could call any time I feel the need to. In the days where there were no GSMs, the doctors in Turkey commonly used to give their patients their home numbers. It's comforting to know you can reach your doctor any time. In Europe, doctors won't give you their private numbers, there is a clean cut between their professional and private lives. In case of emergency, you have to go through the hospital, which then informs your doctor if necessary. Usually, a doctor on call – whom you've never met before – takes care of you. I'm not one of those who like to call their doctors for trivial reasons, I respect private time ex-working hours. I wouldn't call unless I feel it's absolutely necessary. But it's a comfort to me to have my doctor's personal number saved on my cellphone. It has a calming effect for any patient to know they can reach their doctor at any time.

I could never forget the time when I thought I had a urinary tract infection when I was 20 weeks pregnant with the twins and couldn't reach Dr. Markowich for days. I couldn't talk to the doctor herself and I couldn't explain myself very well to her nurse who only spoke French. I was to find out later, through first-hand experience, what a delay of a few days might cost you. I believe the European doctors' policy of withholding their private numbers from their patients hurts the doctor-patient relationship and sometimes complicates it too.

I place the baby's monochromatic sonogram picture and Dr.

Levent's business card happily in my purse and we leave, to meet again in the next month's appointment.

Thursday Market

One Thursday morning, my mother and I decide to take a look around the weekly market, after we drop Matteo off to summer school. Tekirdağ's Thursday market is more fun to me than the funfair. Some find it's torture to go to the market, while I find it very entertaining and distracting. When I lived in Etiler, Istanbul, I used to go to the market in Ulus, where people would come from all around Istanbul and where you could find the garments and accessories of the latest trends simultaneously with, or even before, the shops. I was very interested in the export surplus items from famous brands, I witnessed garments hit the stall in Ulus market at very reasonable prices, of famous brands that I used to see in shops in Spain, Belgium or Britain. The customers rummaging the stalls are delighted when they come across such pieces, and keep turning over the goods piled on the stand in search for more. The Thursday market in Tekirdağ has grown so large that it now runs rings around Ulus market in Istanbul, there is absolutely nothing you cannot find in here; kitchenware, all kinds of gadgets, weird inventions from China, lingerie, pajamas, evening dresses, purses, even dressy high-heels... I've even seen bridal gowns!

The buzz of the market place is energizing, but I'm as cautious as always, walking slowly for 50 yards and then taking a rest. I ask a stallholder permission to sit on their stool, which they never deny. You have to walk around the market streets from one end to the other and rummage every stall to really enjoy the market, but today I confine myself to look around and soak up the atmosphere, I'm grateful for even this much, compared to the time when I was pregnant with Matteo and ordered to stay at home for months.

After my previous pregnancy that I had to spend in bed rest, this pregnancy is pure bliss, I feel free as a bird! I'm now an expert in shopping without wearing myself out, without standing for too long. Three T-shirts; a coffee break; two body suits; two pairs of shorts; a cherry break; two gold fish, one orange and one black; their bowl and their food; a toilet break; and buying fresh fruit and vegetables: all this in one hour! We head back home with bags filled with clothes (almost all of them for Matteo and Submarine#2) and a few pounds of Tekirdağ's famous cherries. I can't get enough of the market place, it's so large you could hardly go around it all if you had a whole day to spend. Sex and the City's Carrie would probably think herself in heaven here and would come up with millions of different combinations for her wardrobe!

"May God Relieve You!"

Whomever I come across in the street will point at my belly and mutter: "May God relieve you!" It's a classical Turkish expression, used for people who are ailing or inflicted with a prison punishment, I find it odd that they use it for expecting mothers as well, as if pregnancy was an ailment or a prison sentence... As I spent my previous pregnancies in Europe, I never heard such phrases, so I'm not familiar with this and find it weird. In Europe, you were more likely to hear people uttering things like "I wish you a healthy pregnancy," or "I hope your baby is well," nothing further. This practice of expressing good wishes to people (even strangers) is very common in Turkey and I normally enjoy it but this "May God relieve you," sounds really unnecessary to me. Well, I have to admit, when you're expecting you are restricted in many ways but it's not a prisoner's life, after all! In old times, the risk of the mother losing her life during delivery was considerably higher, so maybe it made sense then, but I think it's high time for an update, this expression should be removed from the lexicon. I doubt any expectant mother enjoys hearing it.

Keeping Clear of the Sea

"Swimming in the sea is alright but the swimming pool is off limits. There is always a risk of catching an infection even in a clean swimming pool. And when you swim, change out of your wet swimming suit as soon as you come out of the sea, as it may cause a yeast infection in the genital area. Beware of the sun; the best time for expectant mothers to go sun- and sea-bathing is late afternoon." Thus was the advice of my doctor in Brussels, following my cervical cerclage operation. But then, she didn't know about the pollution in Marmara Sea, if she had, she probably would have told me to forget about swimming until delivery.

During pregnancy, when your body temperature is naturally higher, it may be harmful to stay in the sun. Exposure to the sun between 11.00 a.m. and 4.00 p.m. is hazardous for anybody anyway... I find it best to stay in and rest all day. The first week we've arrived in Turkey, some weird jellyfish caught my attention on the beach. Not that I haven't seen jellyfish before, when I was a child, we used to see a lot of clear jellyfish and swim with them around, they were totally harmless, but this kind I've never seen before. They are clear, but there are weird black lines in them, as if they were poisoned by the polluted sea. It turns out I wasn't worried for nothing, when they hit the headlines on TV and in the newspapers in a few days: The pollution in Marmara Sea has created a new breed of jellyfish, which, unlike the ones we used to play with when we were children, are poisonous. The news reporters come to Tekirdağ to film them and show them to their audience, they say you should avoid contact with them. I had doubts about the cleanliness of the sea in the first place, now with the appearance of these nasty jellyfish, I've made up my mind, no matter how I love the sea, I'll have to confine myself to paddling on the shore. It's tormenting to be so close to the sea and not being able to dive in! I ask my doctor in Turkey to be sure, but he's cautious too, "Marmara Sea is polluted," he says, "normally it shouldn't hurt, but it's not worth taking another risk when your pregnancy is risky as it is. If you have to go sea-bathing, you might think of driving to Saroz Bay, the closest Aegean beach to where we are, there you can swim as much as you wish." So, I was right! Apparently, this is to be the first summer I'll be deprived from the pleasure of swimming in the sea ever since I was a baby, I'll have to make do with looking at sea from a distance. They say your life will change completely after you have a baby, I think you don't have to wait until then, the change starts with pregnancy. You start to live with a constant feeling of responsibility and guilt from the day you find out you are pregnant and it goes on after the baby is born!*

---

* My son was used to swimming pools, but it was time to introduce him to the sea, which is always scarier for kids. Children who are not used to the sea find it hard to overcome their fear. So we spent our first week just playing on the sand in the beach. The sea was

The Baby Under Close Watch

Somewhere between the 18th and 22nd week, a special sonogram has to be taken with a different machine by a specialist. Dr. Aret Kamar, my ob-gyn in Istanbul refers me to Dr. Fehmi Yazıcıoğlu, a colleague of his who's a specialist in this field. On the day of our appointment, my father and I prepare to go to Istanbul. Matteo will be staying in the summer house with his grandmother. It takes only about an hour and a half, at most two hours to get there, yet my father has bought us some of Tekirdağ's famous cheese halva and my mother is placing a bag full of plums she's picked from the garden and washed into my purse, so I have something to snack on if I feel a little hungry on the way. And I thought I was good to go with a bottle of water and a book!

The road is nice and quiet, there is next to no traffic, my father drives slowly and carefully, not to rock me. The pleasant journey lasts only as far as the exit from Tekirdağ, as soon as we arrive to the toll booths at the entrance of Istanbul we are faced with the hellish traffic. How come the traffic turns into a right mess past the toll booths when everything was fine just a moment before? I don't understand. I think to myself, I'd probably deliver on the road if I were trying to make it to the hospital for delivery right now. I wonder if anybody has ever given birth in a vehicle in a traffic jam in Istanbul. It seems highly probable to me! Good thing

---

not very attractive anyway, invaded by jellyfish. But on our third week here, the jellyfish finally disappeared and the sea cleared. One day, when the sea was crystal clear, while I was having a walk along the shore, Matteo jumped in the water, encouraged by another kid a little older than he was, and that was the end of his fear of the sea!

we've allowed ample time for the trip. We've left early hoping to stop by our cousin Anıl who has an office in Levent. As the trip stalls, I start to feel tired, so the comfortable couches in Anıl's office make my day. I really need to rest a while, so I lie down on a couch, after asking if it's alright.

I feel a little guilty for having sat upright in the car for hours. After resting for a while, we hit the traffic again to go to our appointment. The doctor's office is in Mecidiyeköy, right across from Profilo Shopping Mall. I may not have been to Mecidiyeköy for years and the last time I've been to Profilo was in 2003, I'm amazed to see how much the place has changed, I cannot recognize the streets, everything has changed, the buildings have been replaced by larger ones, the crowd has grown denser. Even the isolated side alleys are filled with shops. The entrance to Profilo Shopping Mall is almost lost in the crowded ambiance, I can hardly find it. We park the car in Profilo's parking lot and walk through the mall to go out, seeing the café at the entrance floor brings back memories: This is where we met with Cosimo on our first date, which I remember as if it were yesterday...*

... It was the year 2000. My boyfriend and I were going out on our first official date and we'd decided to go see a movie in Profilo Mall, we wanted to see a movie that had won an Oscar award. The movie, of course, was just an excuse to meet, we were eager to see each other. Going to dinner on the first date makes me nervous, it's not fun to eat in front of a man you don't know very well and to whom you want to look attractive, I find it easier to go to a movie. You first have a bite to eat in a café and make small talk to ease into getting to know each other, then you go to the movie and you don't have to talk much, except during the break or at the end, when you comment about the film and decide

when you would like to meet next time. So you don't have to sit facing one another for hours, searching for suitable subjects to talk about and feeling awkward. That's how we'd planned our first date with Cosimo, but sometimes things don't go according to the plan. We were to meet at the café at the entrance floor of the mall to have a cup of coffee before the movie and I got there on time, the first date means the first impression, after all. I sat there waiting for 10 minutes, then 20, then half an hour, but he wouldn't show up! And his cell phone was turned off. I didn't know him very well yet, but somehow I was sure he'd turn up, something must have gone wrong. My heart was divided between leaving, seeing we'd already missed the movie, and waiting a while longer, thinking he could not have stood me up and he'd eventually show up. I decided to hang in there and he finally came, about an hour late! You could see how much stress he'd been through during that last hour while he'd been trying to make it to our rendezvous. He was coming from Maslak, he'd got caught up in that stupid traffic, and he'd had a flat tire, and his cellphone battery had run out, to top it all! He was so sorry and helpless, he apologized sincerely several times. It wasn't possible not to accept his apology or to not believe him. As we'd missed the movie, he invited me to his house to watch one on video tape (yes, those were the days of the video tape). When we got there, he asked me if I would like a hot drink and said he had a lovely jasmine tea. That was just what I needed. A nice, hot cup of jasmine tea, prepared by the man I fancied, on that cold winter night would be perfect, even though it would cause me to stay awake. We sat on a little table made out of dark wood, which he'd bought from a vintage shop in Moscow. He poured the tea he'd steeped in a teapot from China into white cups of a minimalist design. Even his sugar bowl was extraordinary, made of a slab of rock with little holes on top to hold individual sugar cubes. I thought that was just the right guy for me, my house being filled with unusual objects acquired from different places. Many people asked me where I found those, but now I could see I wasn't alone! We took our tea cups and our biscuits to the living room, we picked an Italian movie that'd been recently released from among his collection of video tapes, and started to watch. This man was not like the others, he'd invited me over to watch a movie and here we were, earnestly watching a movie. Not that he didn't want what most men want, he probably did, but I could feel he was happy just to be with me and to share a moment together. We had a great time together that night. It's been nine years since, but we still enjoy having a movie night at home accompanied by jasmine tea and biscuits as we did on our first date.

Dancing Inside My Belly

My little baby has turned to face us. He wants to meet me. He just can't keep still, he keeps moving. It comforts me to see he's fine and healthy, I'm filled with peace as I do everytime I have a sonogram. The doctor, moving the sonogram wand over my belly, starts by examining the baby's brain. He looks at the monochromatic 2-D sections carefully. My father interrupts the silence from time to time, going, "Oh, that's incredible... How amazing... Wow!" The doctor smiles, I feel the need to explain: "It's the first time my father sees such a detailed sonogram, so he's a little excited." My father is elated that he can be near me during my pregnancy, to share every detail. He says it's more exciting to be a granddad than being a dad. Fathers are usually too anxious to enjoy the excitement fully.

The doctor asks me if I can understand the cross-sections,

to which I answer by saying I'm an architect. "Then you would have heard the story of Sinan the Architect," he says, "the way he never drew any plans but described what he had in his mind to the workers by building models." I nod. Honestly, I'd never thought of looking at the sonogram cross-sections from an architect's perspective! The doctor examines each organ; the face, the heart, the lungs, the kidneys, the bladder, the spine and the skeletal system, one by one. He looks at the little heart a little more closely. This is an important exam, as the baby's heart can be viewed in detail only from the 18th to the 20th week. The valves, the veins and arteries are examined. The blood vessels that supply blood to the womb are controlled. The heart exam done while the baby is still in the mother's womb is very useful to determine and possibly prevent the problems that may arise after birth. Prenatal diagnosis allows the planning of the treatment to be applied after birth, it's even possible to perform some surgical operations on babies in the womb, for instance the enlargement of a valve of insufficient size. When I hear of such things, I can't help thinking of my twins (not that I can stop thinking about them at all). If the breakthroughs in modern medicine allow us to do heart surgery on a baby in the womb, how come they couldn't save my twins, whose only problem was loss of amniotic fluid? I just can't wrap my mind around it. I try to accept it as it is and be grateful for the happiness I have now...

It's been almost half an hour since the beginning of the exam, but the baby won't turn his back to us. All the organs have been examined and everything is fine, now it's time to examine the spine. The doctor says we must see the baby's back. He recommends I have a little walk, or go up and down the stairs, as it might help. I do as I'm told, walk around the office, and climb up and down the stairs. When I come back to the exam chair, we see that the baby has turned around, half way if not completely. The doctor manages to take the measurements he needs at this angle thanks to state-of-the-art technology. Apparently, the young one is rather self-indulgent; he can't be bothered to move no matter how much you stair-climbing you do to shake him out of his favorite position. I'm so relieved to find out everything about the baby is normal and he is growing at the average rate. I'm over the moon with happiness, I feel lightened as if a burden had been lifted off my shoulders...

The secretary handed me a sheet of paper and asked me to read and sign it before the procedure. It was an information and consent form about the sonogram, where it says the data about the health of the baby obtained from the procedure may not be a hundred percent accurate, and that accuracy depends largely on the experience and concentration of the doctor who's performing the procedure. It is recommended to save the questions until after the procedure in order not to distract the doctor. But how could an expectant mother keep herself from blurting out question after question when she's faced with weird images on the sonogram screen! I fantasize about having another doctor in the room during the procedure, who would whisper to my ear the facts about what's going on... There is a little box at the bottom of the sheet that the secretary gave me, asking whether I want to have a color picture or a DVD of the sonogram, at an additional fee. You would say it's a photographer's studio! I'm amazed to see how everything is getting more and more costly every year when I come to Istanbul. In the Barcelona and Brussels hospitals, they will put the pictures and DVD's in your file without any additional fees and you don't even have to ask for it. Well, if this is how it is here, we have nothing to do but go along, so we pay the fee and take the picture, and then we say goodbye to the doctor...

Me & My Nightmares

The nightmares that haunted me in every pregnancy I had after my first miscarriages haven't come bothering me for a long time... until tonight. Because I had a healthy pregnancy and delivery the last time and I have a child now, I've been more relaxed this time, convinced that I can deliver a healthy baby. But those nightmares...! I spent the first 24 weeks free from them but now they've come back. My deep rooted fears and unfounded worries keep following me. In my waking hours I make a point of avoiding bad thoughts, quite successfully, too. But they prey upon my sleep. My fears and worries get to me easily when I sleep. I tell them to stay away from me and try to convince myself I'm free from them in this pregnancy, but it doesn't really work. Last night I woke up without a particular reason before dawn, as I do quite often, and couldn't go back to sleep for a while.

When I eventually managed to fall half-asleep, I had a dream, or a nightmare, that felt almost real. I remember praying, during the dream, for it to be a dream! I see myself walking with my huge belly in a crowded street in Şişli, talking to my husband and son, who are having a walk together in a busy street of Brussels, but somehow we happen to be very close to each other, you know what dreams are like. Cosimo tells me to go join them, to which I reply that I have things I need to do here and I can only meet them after I get them done. I'm feeling guilty for having stood on my feet for so long, I'm seized by a sudden fear that something will happen to my baby. Then I feel a wetness in my underwear and a weird sensation in my belly. I go to the toilet in one of the old movie theaters in Osmanbey (Gazi Movie Theater, maybe). My father-in-law is there, too, which surprises me, as he doesn't like to travel much and comes very rarely to see us, he strokes his grandchild over my belly. I go to the toilet, it's strange and dirty place, with old style squat toilets (that you still come across quite often in Turkey) in a row without any separating wall between them, so everybody just goes openly. Even during the dream it seems strange. I see a young girl, with lengths of umbilical cord hanging down from her private parts, she's weeping and crying, she's lost her baby. It's an image like those in extra-terrestrial creature movies; the girl's naked body is covered in a weird, gooey substance, she is helpless, I feel very sorry for her but I cannot do anything to help. I look around for a free toilet and check my underwear, there seems to be no problem, I just have a discharge, but I also feel the baby is gone down very low and is engaged, it feels as if my cerclage sutures have ruptured. "What if the baby comes too early," I worry, "we're only in the 24th week yet, he is not supposed to come, I have to keep him in there! What if I lose him, what am I going to do?" But then I think of Matteo, I'm grateful to have him, and this thought puts my mind at ease. I can't stop thinking of the girl in the toilet, I think to myself I'd better call my doctor...

Then I wake up, soaked in sweat, to Matteo's voice calling me, and I sigh in relief to realize it was only a dream. I had spicy food last night, I guess that's what caused me to have bad dreams. Thanks to my son, I wake up to a lovely day, but I have a hard time shaking off the effect of the life-like dream. I splash cold water on my face to help myself wake up.

We lie on the couch in the living room with Matteo, as we do every morning, to hug and kiss and tickle each other, and we make a Skype call to Cosimo. We like to say good morning to each other as we begin each day. As Italy is an hour behind us, Cosimo is usually rather sleepy when we are wide awake and energetic. Matteo's energy helps his daddy wake up, even from a long distance. We blow each other kisses over the computer screen. Afterwards, we go out to the garden to give our dog Çakır his breakfast, and then I prepare us a wholesome, organic breakfast: fresh milk and eggs from the farm, cheese and butter from the village, homemade jam, honey from the bees in our field, tomatoes, bell peppers, cucumbers from the garden, bread baked at home and fresh baked simit that my father has bought from the baker's, which we devour in good appetite. And so my son makes me forget about the nightmare I've had.

Technology as a Remedy for Yearning

I wish we could be in two places at once or clone ourselves! The only thing I miss in my life at this moment is my husband. It's so hard to be separated from your loved one, especially in a time where your hormones go crazy, like pregnancy... Yes, Cosimo and I did make this decision together. We thought it was the best way both for me and the baby, and our son. My husband was to start in his new position in Italy soon and it didn't make sense for me and

Matteo to stay in Brussels and wait for the move. Furthermore, I had a special pregnancy and had to take care of myself, I needed help for the care of our son. Coming to live with my parents for the rest of my pregnancy was the perfect and most practical solution. Cosimo could get used to his new post, find a house, move in, and we would go back to him soon after the birth, when the house would be ready.

Cosimo and I often read each other's mind and soul, it's as if we communicate telepathically. Once I sent him an e-mail when I missed him dearly, telling him I was making penne with eggplant sauce for Matteo and how I wished he was there with us – it turned out he was writing to me at the very same moment to tell me how he missed us and how he longed for the day where we would come together and he could embrace the three of us. That happens to us very often, we think and feel the same way at the same moment, Cosimo's emotional intelligence is very strong and our mentalities are very compatible.

Last year we used to spend almost 24 hours a day together while he worked from home and couldn't stand being separated for even a few hours, but now he is so far away from us... still, our hearts are with him.

Today is Father's Day! We will not be able to hug and greet him, but at least we have the technology that allows us to make a video call and to blow him kisses over the camera. My son and I are devout Skype users, we log into our Skype account before we go to bed, we place my laptop by the bedside, and Cosimo can tell Matteo his bedtime story. They blow each other kisses and say good night over the camera, and Matteo goes to sleep in peace, having seen his father.

I've also familiarized my parents with the Internet, they've started to use a computer after the age of 60, for the sake of their grandson. They know now that they can always see and talk to him even when we are away from each other. They may not be able to hug and kiss him but they can at least see him, which alleviates the sorrow of separation.

To be away from my husband is something I'm not used to, it turns out I missed missing him! Missing someone is nice when you know you'll end up seeing them again!*

Hooray, Daddy is Here!

So far with being separated, I'll soon be united with my darling husband, and my son with his dear daddy! When I see the way the two of them look at each other I burst into tears. Matteo cries

---

* Every expectant mother needs a husband like Cosimo. When I was pregnant with Matteo, I was told to stay in bed all day, as a precautionary measure, so I was supposed to spend the whole day lying on the couch except going to the bathroom or taking a shower. Cosimo was always by my side when he wasn't working, he waited on me hand and foot, he kept watching the baby daily, he accompanied me to my fortnightly doctor's appointments, he became my private Italian chef and cooked very special dishes following world-famous chefs' recipes, so I got to try sophisticated Italian dishes for the first time. He even tended my personal care when I needed him to, he followed my pregnancy closely and kept an Excel file that he updated weekly, and took photos of my belly every month. He made it easy and pleasant for me to go through my homebound pregnancy.

"Yaşasın, baba geldi*!" when he sees his dad, surprising us all with his Turkish. We kiss, and hug, and kiss again, united in a tight embrace. Matteo is all over his dad, either on his lap or on his back, and won't leave him until bedtime, he's literally stuck to him. He looks at him admiringly and doesn't stop smiling for one moment. There is a common saying in Turkish, which means "May God never separate those who love each other," which I used to find too melancholy but now I know I'll never look down on those who use it.

I've missed everything about my husband, even the way he strokes my belly... As his affectionate hand touches my belly I'm filled with peace, I feel as if I've been lightened with his arrival. The soft touch of peace embraces me all over, I'm with the person who is the love of my life, its essence, its meaning, I'm sure my baby feels it inside my belly. From the fifth month on, the babies start hearing the voices and noises outside the womb. After they are born, they can recall the voices they've heard while in the womb and calm down when they hear those familiar voices. Our little one cannot hear his dad's voice much, except when we talk on the Internet every morning and every night. I hope the baby hears it, too. When he's born, it's going to take a while for him to get used to his dad, but I hope he won't be a stranger to him all together!**

*Cosimo's father was away too when his mother was pregnant with him. His mother had to raise her children almost single handedly, which must explain the distant relationship between my husband and his father. His father Attilyo was a seaman, and it wasn't easy for him to build himself a family as he was away at the sea most of the time.

---

* Hooray, daddy's here!

He and Agnese grew up together in the same town. First someone thought they were well-suited to each other, Attilyo had liked her for some time anyway. They were lucky, they fell for one another, and they got married (they are soon to celebrate their 50th anniversary). After the wedding, they spent their first night as a married couple together. (My mother-in-law says it was almost unthinkable for a couple to sleep together before getting married in those days. Southern Italy was strictly Catholic and sex was taboo, the bride had to be a virgin, but it didn't matter how experienced the groom was. A lot has changed since then and the first night is no longer an issue in Italy, but in many places on the world, and in Turkey, it's still a requirement that the bride be virginal, which is why hymenoplasty, that is, hymen repair surgery, is so common in Arabic countries and in Turkey. I don't quite understand who's fooling who! Unfortunately, this is where we stand in the 21st century!) My mother-in-law got pregnant with her first child, Cosimo, that very first night! The next day the newlywed couple was separated as Attilyo had to go set sail, not to come back for six months! It's an irritating story for those who struggle for years to have a baby, but this was how fertile women were back then. It makes sense, of course. It's easier to conceive when you are younger and live a life without stress. Everything is getting easier but we make things harder for ourselves for reasons we can't change much. Cosimo's mother saw her husband only once or twice during her pregnancy, he was away at sea even on the day of her delivery. When you are on a nautical voyage, you cannot just come back when you wish to! An airplane pilot could just jump on a plane and come home, but it's not the same with a seaman. Cosimo had not seen much of his father while he was growing up, he was almost a fatherless child. His mother had to fill in for him, too. It's a good thing she's a strong and strict character. They had their second son in four years, and their daughter eight years later. The second boy wasn't any luckier than Cosimo with regard to having their father with them, but a girl was born after their father had retired and therefore had the opportunity to develop a better, closer relationship with their father.

How I Become a Favoured Patient... Thanks to a Bottle of Italian Wine

My doctor in Tekirdağ is a real traveler. I guess he's spending all his spare time traveling the world. I noticed the heap of travel magazines on the table in the reception area the first time I was in his office. He has been to many places in Italy and acquired much knowledge of its regional food and wines. When he meets my husband, he asks him where in Italy he is from, and when Cosimo tells him he's from Puglia, he quickly recalls the information he has of the region, and says, "They are famous with their white wine, aren't they?" I think to myself he's asking the right question to the right guy. Although he doesn't drink much, Cosimo is so knowledgeable about wine that he can go on for hours like a wine connoisseur. After they have a short chat about wines, the doctor tells Cosimo how lucky he is to be Italian, to which Cosimo replies, as a great fan of Turkey, that we are the lucky ones to be Turkish and to live in such a lovely country. Finally we agree that we're all very lucky.

Before the sonogram, we talk about my pregnancy and the stage we're in. The doctor asks me if I have any complaints. I say I feel some pain at the right side of my belly if walk a little too much (of course, what I call too much would hardly be over 100 yards, I'm really cautious about being on my feet). He says it's completely normal, as the baby grows the womb slides to the right and pushes on the other organs, and, of course, it might be flatulence, too. He tells me to stop taking the vitamin supplements except folic acid and iron, and to start taking magnesium daily and cod liver oil capsules every other day. Omega fatty acids found in cod liver oil is good for the baby's brain development. He also asks me to have a urine test this month. And then comes the grimmest moment of the appointment, where I have to step on the scale: I've gained 5 pounds and a half in a month. My doctor is not happy about it, neither am I, but I know why, it's because of all the watermelon I've been eating to fight the summer heat, and all the fresh corn boiled in huge pots I can't resist. I'm supposed to gain 3 to 4.5 pounds per month at most. Although I know how many pounds an expectant mother is supposed to gain throughout her pregnancy, I ask him once more, to which he replies it varies from woman to woman, but it should ideally be between 20 to 30 pounds. "Not everybody has to gain weight," he says, "although it's exceptional, I had a patient who actually lost weight during pregnancy yet gave birth to a healthy baby of 9 pounds, but she was actually over 220 pounds to start with." It was an exceptional case, the doctor gave her a special diet, which allowed the baby to gain weight while she lost it. The female body is astonishing, you learn something new every day. He tells me to watch what I eat.

So, it wasn't for no reason that I couldn't fit into my clothes and underwear any more, apparently I lost control! Cosimo teases me, saying "We will not be able to take Demi Moore shots of you if you go on like this!" My husband who loves photography took beautiful black and white photos of me with my huge, naked belly, on the seventh month of my pregnancy with Matteo, throughout which I only gained 29 pounds, which didn't show that much. Especially my face was almost the same as it was before I got pregnant. I consider myself lucky in that aspect, even when I gain a lot of weight, it doesn't show much on my face. As I spent that pregnancy in bed rest, I didn't exert myself and I didn't feel the urge to eat much. But I'm more active this time, therefore my metabolism is higher and I need to eat. Add to that the irresistible summery foods and my hearty appetite... no surprise the pounds keep piling up. I promised my husband and my doctor, and myself, to be careful about what I eat until the end of my pregnancy, and I will!

✦

And now, the happiest moment of the exam, where I see my baby son on the sonogram screen. He is turning around, spinning, tumbling, standing upside down, and doing all kinds of acrobatics in his private little pool. This time he won't turn to face us, we can only see a little bit of his face from the side. The doctor thinks his head looks like my husband's, who says the resemblance is only because he and the baby are both bald and makes us laugh. I'm so happy looking at the image on the screen, I could watch him for hours. My darling husband holds my hand tight as he does every time he's with me during a sonogram. His warm hands warm my heart and give me courage. The doctor carefully takes the measurements he needs to take, I don't want to talk much and distract him when he needs to focus but I can't help asking for the baby's weight and height. He's gained 4.5 pounds since last month. The pounds I've gained weren't good news but this is. In my mind, I say, "Way to go, my baby, go on, grow up, and let what I eat feed you." You cannot measure exactly how tall a baby is while he's still in the womb, but it can be estimated from the length of the thigh bone. Our baby seems to be taller than average, the doctor says he'll be a tall man. All the measurements look alright, the cerclage and the cervix are intact. I sigh in relief as I do after every exam. We take the picture of the Submarine Number 2 that the doctor hands us, we say goodbye and leave the doctor's office happy as clams in mud. It's our last day together, after which we will not be seeing each other for 35 days. We drop in my brother's café before going home and have drink of homemade mint lemonade. Lemonade is the most popular drink in Turkey this summer, the stores are flooded with different brands of lemonade, but none of them compares to my brother's.

In my next visit to the doctor's, I bring him a gift of a bottle of Prosecco, the famous wine of the Veneto region of Italy. He's delighted. He asks me to translate the label. I tell him it's a good wine to have with seafood and hors d'oeuvres. He thanks me and says, "This wine puts you on the list of most favorite patients," and we laugh...

I take a urine sample to a laboratory I've heard is good, to have the test done. The result shows a lot of bacterial activity. And I've been so careful, I haven't set foot in the sea or the swimming pool, I've even been careful with the water I use for personal cleansing, I've mostly avoided public toilets, I'm so surprised I cannot believe the result. Now, that's just what I needed! A pregnant woman can never breathe easy, we are overwhelmed with tests and exams. During my mother's time, pregnancy was calmer, more relaxed. They didn't have all these tests and sonograms that show you everything, they used to listen to the baby's heartbeat once a month, which indicated the baby was alive, and that was it. I call my doctor, who tells me to have the test repeated in a different laboratory, and to have an additional test done to indicate which antibiotics I should use. This time, the result comes clean, no bacteria, I don't know what to believe anymore. The doctor recommends I drink plenty of water, and I'm happy I got through without taking any drug. I ask him what a urinary tract infection during pregnancy might cause, he says it might even lead to preterm delivery and therefore one cannot be too careful... The latest research studies show that over 70 percent of preterm deliveries are due to bacterial infections of the reproductive organs. Here's another issue to stress about. You never know till it happens to you; there's so much around us that threatens the baby's health, when I think it's safe and sound inside my belly. If I start to think about it, I know I'll never be able to stop. I'd better not dwell too long on this issue, otherwise I'll fall prey to anxiety again...

The Ideal Birthday

We are going to Istanbul to meet our baby on week 25. We've timed our appointment to coincide with my birthday and taken two days off our daily routine for the trip. I am hoping to stay in a nice hotel with a view on the Bosphorus and have some time alone with my husband after the appointment. And I've been celebrating my birthday in Istanbul for years, it's almost like a tradition now. I put a glamorous maternity dress in my little suitcase, along with my make-up and toiletries. We pick our lunch bags containing slices of mother's delicious minced meat and eggplant pie and some tiny, crisp cucumbers from father's greenhouse. We put Matteo in mother's care and leave for Istanbul. It's only a short drive from Tekirdağ to Istanbul, but I'm rather fussy when I'm pregnant. I feel I've been sitting upright too long in the car and worn myself out, so I want to go to the hotel to have a lie down before the appointment. I've been suffering from back pain for some time and it's been getting more severe lately. My husband obliges his pregnant wife without complaining, saying "There's no point in going early anyway, they'll keep us waiting as they always do." I've been criticizing him for going to doctor's appointments ahead of time for years, we've spent countless minutes in reception areas and hospital hallways waiting to be admitted, I'm glad he has finally come to his senses after nine years!

When an Expectant Mother Falls...

There are few hotels in Istanbul from the roof of which you can see the historical peninsula, the Golden Horn, and the Bosphorus at once. The view is so exciting! The roof of The Marmara Pera, with its lovely panorama, is the ideal and cool place to relax in the overwhelming summer heat. It's the 20th of July, 2009, I'll celebrate my 39th birthday when the clock strikes midnight, if I can stay up that late. Every birthday is special but I guess this one means more to me as it's the last of my 30s. My husband and I will be staying at The Marmara Pera to indulge ourselves...

The doctor's office is in Gümüşsuyu, as the hotel is on our way we just drop in to leave our luggage and to have a rest. I'm wearing leather sandals. As soon as I set my foot out of the car, I step on a slanted area of the road, with the asphalt molten in the sun, slip and lose my balance. Luckily, I fall neatly on my backside. My husband and the hotel attendants waiting at the door panic, everybody rushes to help get the pregnant woman up on her feet. I'm totally alright and hurt nowhere, except my big toe that rubbed against the asphalt, but I'm really scared. I rush into bed and lie down still as a rock, listening to my baby kicking in my belly. Cosimo keeps asking me how I feel – although I hurt nowhere except my big toe, I'm deeply worried, I can't wait to get to the doctor's and see the baby on the sonogram. Most women tumble at least once during their pregnancy, it happens to almost all expectant mothers, as the huge belly throws the body off balance. It's scary even to think of falling but it happens...

The hallways in the hospital are hang with pictures of babies. The card I sent from Brussels when Matteo was born is up on the billboard, it's nice to see it there. It's our first meeting with my dear doctor after a long while, but we haven't lost touch, I've kept him informed of the events in my life through phone calls and e-mail messages. I give him a brief summary, as he has hundreds of patients. Dr. Aret too thinks it's unexceptional that I got pregnant without therapy. He reminds me that I gave birth to my son through vaginal delivery and asks me how I feel about it this time. I say I'd like to have a vaginal delivery again, with an epidural.*

---

* I want to be clear about delivery. I know as a fact that ob-gyns and expectant mothers in Turkey are totally pro-C-section. The C-section mania of the Turkish is known even in the hospitals in Europe. I for one am against C-section by choice, without a medical necessity. Some women, although they are capable of delivering naturally, feel it's easier to deliver via C-section. Expectant mothers wish for everything to be over and done with without pain, so they could hold their baby when they come to. But the postpartum

And, my baby son appears on screen! How comforting it is to see him, even though it's only an image. My doctor points out that the cervical cerclage is a little too low. He thinks the suture should be higher, closer to the baby. I'm now used to the fact that all doctors may not see eye to eye on various matters and I've come to accept it. I keep my cool, and ask him what it might lead to. He says there's nothing to worry about but I should take frequent sonograms to be on the safe side.

I'm happy with the idea of being closely monitored, and used to it too, as my doctor in Brussels used to see me every other week... Now it's time to watch the baby move inside my belly, the best part of the exam to me... My little one is doing somersaults in his private pool. He stops for a moment, and – unbelievable as it is – turns to face us fully, there is a smile-like expression on his face. The doctor wiggles the sonogram wand and catches this rare moment in print. The picture surprises even the nurse, who says we're lucky he turned to face us. His nose and mouth seem to look like his big brother's, we can see almost all his facial features clearly. Long live technology! Only thirty years ago, when my mother was pregnant with my brother, all we could hear was his heartbeat, but now we can see a baby inside the womb through

---

period is harder. After all, C-section is a surgical operation, and you end up with an incision on your abdomen, how easy do you think it would be to hold a baby when you have that? Sometimes the letdown of milk can take some time, and it can take even longer in case of a C-section. The babies are generally impatient and get very irritable when they suckle and no milk comes, so you are compelled to feed them with a bottle, which puts a stop to breastfeeding before it starts. Most lazy babies get used to the bottle at once and refuse the breast for good.

a sonogram. It's true that modern life deprives us of many things but it brings a lot in return, we cannot complain...

Dr. Aret carefully takes the head and abdomen circumference measurements, and concludes that everything is fine and I should stick to my slow pace, he hands the picture of Submarine Number 2 to his dad, and we take leave, to come back in a month...

Cihangir: An Unobstructed View of Istanbul at a Very Short Distance

It's only 7.00 p.m. The sun is still hot but it's already dinner time for me... I ask my husband if he would like to go to Doğa Balık, a nice fish restaurant that we both like. He likes the idea... We can have a nice fish with a healthy side of Aegean herbs, and enjoy the view of Istanbul and the Bosphorus that we've been missing. It's been years since we last ate there. It's only a short distance from Gümüşsuyu to Cihangir and it would be a nice walk in such a lovely summer evening, but I don't feel comfortable walking when I'm expecting, let alone walking uphill. A cab stops, I ask the driver if he could take us to Cihangir. Quite predictably, he replies that it's too short a distance, with a sour face. But when I tell him that I'm pregnant and not supposed to walk much, his attitude changes immediately, and he says: "Oh, sure, just jump in, I'll take you there." That's the spirit! I love that about my countrymen, I think to myself how nice it is to be pregnant.

Once in Doğa Balık, we order a platter of hors d'oeuvres consisting of Aegean herbs and an octopus salad that we wolf down with a sip of Efes beer. Then we order angler fish, I love fish and try to have it on the menu at least once or twice a week. I consumed so much fish when I was expecting Matteo, which may be the reason he loves it, too. I often hear mothers saying their children won't eat fish and they have to give them fish oil capsules to compensate. We've never had this problem, Matteo will devour a sea bass and a half on his own.

The restaurant is located at the roof terrace of a hotel, from where we enjoy the view of Istanbul and the Bosphorus and take plenty of photos like tourists. Since we've been living overseas, we've felt more like tourists each time we come back to Istanbul. When you're here only for a short while, you can't get enough of Istanbul. This is exactly how we feel at the moment, we are happy to be here. We decide to go and watch the sunset from the roof terrace of our hotel, and fly from one roof to the other...

The secret of the geographical beauty of Istanbul is the hills on which she's been built. If it was a flat city, you could see the Bosphorus only from the its shore, whereas as it is, it surprises you with a different perspective every time you look at it from a different hill top. The roof terrace of the hotel is brimming with tourists, both Turkish and foreign, wishing to watch the sunset. We pick ourselves a spot at the bar with an unobstructed view of the historical peninsula. Lots of photos, lots of kisses, a great view, and a lot of wind! One of the strange things about Istanbul is that, while you are overwhelmed with the heat during the day, at night you will shiver in the cool wind. That's the beauty of this city. In many metropolises in the world you will suffocate in the July heat, while the cool night breath of the Bosphorus comforts Istanbul. I'm prepared, I have a scarf and my husband with me, I wrap myself up and cuddle against him, to guard my baby and myself from the wind. But when you are pregnant, your hormones burn like an oven inside your body and you cannot stand any exposure to heat from outside, that's why it's not fun to be pregnant in summer. My husband calls me a 'human heater' because of my high body temperature.

Since I'm pregnant, I need to get up from my seat quite often, as sitting for a long time gives me a backache. Bar chairs aren't comfortable anyway. We decide to go to our room to relax and go on taking in the view in our comfy couch against the window. For a moment, I remember how I used to celebrate my birthdays, with a party of at least 30 of my best friends, at home or in a hip venue, dancing like crazy till dawn. Pregnancy changes your body's rhythm and your lifestyle, the best way I can think of to spend my birthday now is to lie down comfortably in my bed, have some pillow talk with my husband, chat with a close friend or two on the phone, and to sleep... During pregnancy, your motto becomes "Sleep, more sleep!" I've been there before, so I know very well, besides, everybody keeps telling me to sleep while I can, as I'll be missing those days once the baby arrives. The first time, I didn't heed the warnings, thinking I could always sleep while the baby slept, but you understand it's not all that easy once you get there. Well, just wait and see, but until then, sleep as much as you can!

There's still an hour to go before midnight but my friends are impatient, they've already started calling to celebrate my birthday. Two of my girlfriends call one after the other to give me their best wishes. I take a warm shower, as I do almost every night throughout my pregnancy, as the water massaging my neck and my back helps me sleep better. But sometimes I wake up in the middle of the night and stay awake for a long time. I've heard of other pregnant women with sleep issues. It's unavoidable to lose sleep in the last months of pregnancy as you get really heavy and cannot find a comfortable sleeping position with your huge belly. But then, there are those like me who lose sleep because they're worried about losing their baby from the very beginning of their pregnancy. Since I'm so preoccupied by my worries, I find it hard to get quality sleep. Add the hormones and the summer heat on top of all that, and you can say goodbye to your zzzs.

When I asked my doctor in Brussels what I could do about my sleeping problem, she'd recommended me to take a warm shower before going to bed. Don't ask Belgian doctors to prescribe you drugs, they won't do that unless really necessary, which is why natural therapies are very established and widely used in Belgium and other northern countries. While Cosimo is searching for a good movie on TV, I go in the shower to prepare myself for bed. When I come back, I find a black case on the pillow, with a note tucked underneath: a birthday surprise from my husband, I cannot believe it! Every year we go shopping for my birthday present together since he is worried about making the wrong choice and getting me something I won't like, this year we haven't had the opportunity to do it, and naturally I didn't expect a gift. His coming from Italy to be with me on my special day is the greatest gift to me, I didn't expect anything else. This comes as a surprise, which makes it even more exciting. My shy husband shuts himself into the bathroom to leave me alone while I'm reading the romantic note he's written. I think to myself it did him good to be away from me for 49 days, it jogged his imagination and allowed him to pick a gift he thought would suit me. It's a hand-made necklace of Murano beads, the clear, white glass beads look so neat and dainty on my neck; it really reflects my style. I love it. I like almost anything that my husband selects for me anyway, he has a refined taste. As my mother will say when she'll see the necklace, Italian men have a way with gifts. I don't mean to offend Turkish men, but that's the truth...

We cuddle and kiss again. I say, "See, it wasn't that hard to give me a surprise," he smiles bashfully. We go to sleep in a hug, happy and peaceful at the end of a long and tiring day... Tomorrow will be the first day of my new age, I have to be in good shape. I plan on sleeping till late in the morning, considering my little alarm clock of a son who wakes me up at seven o'clock sharp every morning is not here. But my biological clock wakes me up at the very same time I'm used to waking up every day. Also, the baby is very active early in the morning, kicking and turning inside my belly. I hope he won't be an early bird like his big brother and will let mommy sleep till late. As soon as I'm awake, I feel I'm starving, and snack on the fruit the hotel brought in the room for my birthday.

It's six in the morning, I watch Istanbul wake up and come to life. An odd car or two go over the Haliç Bridge, the boat trips are about to start in Eminönü Docks... The pink and red hues of the rising sun reflect on the Bosphorus, the morning air is nice and fresh, and I've missed waking up in Istanbul. Submarine Number 2 has finished his morning workout and I get hopeful of going back to sleep, but I wake up again at eight, this time with text messages on my cell phone. It's friend of mine from Italy, I don't know how she does it but she's always the first to celebrate my birthday in the morning. I'm not a really a morning person anyway, and since my son's arrival I've been dedicating my mornings to my family: if you are an expectant mother suffering from morning sickness or a mother whose child keeps nagging you for this and for that, how would you get down to writing birthday messages first thing in the morning? I can write mine only in the tiny breaks I can get during the day, in toilet breaks or after my son goes to bed, I'm grateful if I can get them done before the day is over. Perhaps I don't put pen to paper to write letters or birthday cards like I used to do, but I still keep in touch with my friends all over the world thanks to the Internet.

When you are pregnant, people pamper you even more than usual. We've been celebrating my birthday for two days. Cosimo spares nothing to please me. My parents call to ask me if I want anything special for tonight's dinner. I ask my father for a barbecue and my mother for some hors d'oeuvres. We are going to have a barbecue party, accompanied by a bottle of Prosecco wine Cosimo has brought from Venice to celebrate my birthday. I don't want to wear myself out. At the end of the exam yesterday, the doctor said, "Don't you forget the limitations, thinking you are fine, or I'll order you to bed till the end of your pregnancy," and I promised him I wouldn't, but you just can't leave Istanbul without taking a tour of the Bosphorus and having a cup of coffee in Aşk Kafe, the venue of so many good memories! With Cosimo's approval, we go on a drive along the Bosphorus with my friend Sibel. We take a pleasant break in Aşk Kafe. Elif, my sweet friend from university, calls to celebrate my birthday, and I invite her over. She comes and joins us in a flash. It's been a long time since we last saw each other, we hug and kiss, we're elated. It's so good to see old friends. It's hard to be far away, I miss them so much. Istanbul drains your energy, especially when you're pregnant... I have no strength left at all. The last two days have been too busy for my slow pregnancy pace, it's high time I go back to my quiet haven in Tekirdağ...

A Name for the Baby

It's a tough job to find a name for a baby... I'm sure every international couple goes through the same muddle. It's relatively easier for Spanish, Italian, French or Greek couples as there are dozens of names that are used commonly in both partners' languages. It's harder for a Turkish-Italian couple like us. I haven't come across a single name that's common to both our native tongues, there are a few that have a counterpart with the same sound in the other language, but their meanings and spellings are totally different. For instance, the Turkish name Can sounds a lot like Gian in Italian, but Gian is never used alone, it's always followed by a second name, such as Gianfranco. I don't like such long names, they feel a little outdated. I prefer mono- or disyllabic names. Matteo's meaning, a gift from God, fits my situation exactly, we waited for him for years. He is the greatest gift we could have ever been given in life. The sound is also nice, it's very charismatic. It's easy for the Turkish to spell and pronounce, as it has a phonetic spelling; in fact it's a name that wouldn't cause any trouble in no part of the world. I like this idea, my son will be comfortable with his name wherever he goes. He started travelling overseas at the age of five months, he has travel lovers for parents, so I guess it's a sure thing that he will be a traveler in his own right when he grows up.

It may sound like an easy job to name a baby, but it's a great responsibility. You must find a name that, first of all, he himself will like. I find it wrong to give a child a name that will not match their physical appearance. If you name a boy of small, slender build Aslan (that means Lion in Turkish), for instance, the weight of the name will crush him. In recent years, there is a trend for fancy names. Especially world-famous stars give their children names like Apple or Pear, or names out of story books. If they want to be extraordinary, that's nobody's business, but what did those children do to deserve it? They'll always be people's laughing stock with their uncommon, hard to pronounce names. I've always liked Latin names. Matteo was one of the first names I came up with, and my husband liked it too, so we decided on our firstborn's name without any hesitation. But we're having a hard time finding a name for our second son. He will be here in a few months but we've still not picked a name that we both like. He doesn't like the ones I propose, and vice versa. Some of our name choices seem quite close the each other's but we haven't come to a full agreement on any name yet. We still call my little son by the name of Submarine Number 2. I'm hoping to find him a fitting name judging by his looks in the sonograms to come...

Can a Pregnant Woman Not Wear Thin Clothes in the Summer?

The baby's arriving in November. Most of my pregnancy takes place in summer. I find it hard to be pregnant in summer, the only good part being the freedom to wear thin clothes. My mother too had a summer pregnancy once, and there was no air conditioning then, poor mom... As I was telling her about something funny that happened to me recently, I found out she had a similar thing happen to her back then; this tells me that clothing is still taboo for the Turkish in many ways, after all these years. You feel it even more in little towns. It's my 30th week, I'm seven months pregnant, and I have a doctor's appointment around noon. It's August, the town is burning, and the temperature is almost 90 degrees. I'm wearing one of the outfits I find most comfortable in this heat; a white cotton shirt and a long, black, pleated cotton skirt that hugs my belly with its broad elastic waist band, free and easy.

I like to wear a skirt to sonogram appointments, so I don't have to strip; you can just pull your skirt up. Everything goes well during the exam, I see my baby in the sonogram, I'm relieved to hear the doctor say all is well, and I'm on my way home, happy as a clam. Walking toward my car, I go past a café, with tables on the curb. It's noon, on one of the tables two youngsters are having pizza and talking, on another one a woman in her 40s is having lunch on her own, she's eating her food heartily, maybe a little hurriedly, apparently she's got little time.

I leave the café behind and I'm about to reach my car in about 20 yards that I hear a voice behind me, calling, "Excuse me, madam." I turn around, it's the lady in the café, scurrying towards me. I say "Yes," trying to make her out. Breathlessly, she says, "Sorry, I just wanted to warn you, I think you may have forgotten to put on your underskirt." There you have it. Making an effort not to be rude, I say, "Thank you for your warning, but I haven't. I like to wear this skirt as it is." A similar incident happened to my mother 30 years ago, when she wore a dress made of Şile cloth* to a monthly prenatal visit. After the exam, the nurse assisting my mother gives her the once-over and says, "You'd better wear an underskirt, you can see through your skirt." I guess those who make such comments don't know a thing about being pregnant;

---

* Şile cloth is a light, gauzy cotton fabric made in Şile district of Istanbul.

an underskirt means an extra layer of clothing, and usually made of synthetic fabric, too.

Mercurial Questions

Now in the seventh month of my pregnancy, I've left most dark thoughts and worries behind and I'm in a lighthearted mood, which may be due to the fact that we're nearing the happy ending or to my conscious positive thinking efforts.

As I'm going to my doctor's appointment in Istanbul, I'm filled with a feeling of confidence that I cannot describe. This time I'm accompanied by my brother Can. We arrive in Istanbul after a nice drive. It's a hot August day, but luckily there is a breeze in Istanbul today. The café in The Marmara has been one of my favorite meeting spots with my friends, it's now called Kitchenette but it's the same venue as it was before. We meet with the girls for luncheon before my appointment, Sibel, Umut, Ornella and I talk about babies, and men, and fashion, and Istanbul venues, and the country's economics, trying to squeeze it all in one hour. That's how women are, not only we are able to multi-task, we can also multi-talk!

Sibel accompanies me to my appointment. We take a cab from Taksim Square to Gümüşsuyu, a distance of 200 yards at most, but the sympathetic cab drivers are willing to take a pregnant woman anywhere she asks, without complaining. I often witness how pregnant woman are treated with respect and care and I like it very much. I've decided to spend the rest of my life with a pillow on my belly.

I've been to so many doctor's exams for years that I should

have had the answers to all possible questions, but pregnancy is such a complicated topic that you come up with new questions every day. I've covered all the general topics and I'm down to fine detail now. The major issue in today's appointment is mercury, which amuses my doctor very much. I've known Dr. Aret Kamar for over three years, he kindly listened to me and answered my questions every time I called him, no matter from where on earth. In my pregnancy with Matteo, I started fertility treatment with him in Istanbul and went on with another doctor in Brussels, still he provided long-distance support throughout my pregnancy over the phone. He's helped me gradually overcome my fears with his comforting and reassuring words.

He says, "God bless you, Nur! I've heard all kinds of questions in years but this is the first time I'm hearing this. Where did you come up with this?" I reply I keep reading non-stop, books, magazines, Internet articles, any material I can lay my hands on. I love fish and seafood, and I've been consuming a lot of fish during my pregnancy as I heard it was good, but recently I've read somewhere that too much fish may be harmful as it may cause mercury accumulation in the body, which has made me wonder whether it might hurt the baby and I've decided I'd discuss the issue with him.

I keep surprising and amusing him with my questions. They say long lived fish such as salmon, tuna and mackerel are prone to heavy metal build-up in their flesh and they might be harmful if consumed in large quantities. I had a lot of salmon the other day so I couldn't help worrying and I had to ask. Dr. Aret teases my worries away. The exam goes on with jokes, I relax and find myself lying on the sonogram chair, looking at my baby. The doctor knows me very well. I seem to be over my fear of sonograms, I take pleasure in seeing my baby, my handsome son inside my belly. I can see his profile clearly, we decide with the doctor that he has a large nose. As the baby grows, the lines become clearer. I ask about his weight and height, to which the doctor replies by saying that I shouldn't worry about that, that anything from 5.5 to 9 pounds is alright. He goes on to say we cannot measure exactly how tall the baby is. The prenatal measurements of weight are not real measurements but estimations, which help assess the course of the pregnancy and the health of the baby, and that's enough for us.

As We Near the Happy Ending

As the weeks fly and we near the end, the excitement soars. I have mixed feelings, on one hand I want this pregnancy to be over, on the other I'm sad that it's soon going to. It's great to carry my baby inside my belly, to know that his little heart is beating inside me.

The last months of my pregnancy increase my anticipation and decrease my fears... When I was expecting Matteo, I didn't worry much about making it to the hospital when I'd go into labor, as we lived at 10 minutes' distance to the hospital. Even if my contractions started of my waters broke while I was alone at home, I knew I could always call a cab and get to the hospital in 10 minutes. But the idea of going to Istanbul for delivery scares me. I'm sure every expectant woman living in Istanbul experiences the fear of getting stuck in traffic and not being able to reach the hospital on time. Not everybody can live in the vicinity of their hospital of preference but distance is definitely a factor to consider when selecting a hospital.

I've got a fear rooted in my heart from my previous pregnancies; the fear of my waters breaking early... That's the first question I ask the doctor in each appointment: "Is the amniotic fluid level alright? Is the cervix intact?" I've become quite an expert in that matter. The distance between the cervix and the baby's head decreases as the delivery comes nearer. After the 36th week onwards, there's nothing to worry about, you are very close to term, the baby's development is practically complete; it's alright even if he comes a little early. Of course, we aim at having the baby reach the term of 40 weeks inside the womb.

❧

I'm not really scared of labor pain, or being hurt, or anesthesia. No doubt, I owe this at least partially to having delivered before and seen it's no big deal. But I wasn't afraid of giving birth even before my first delivery. My pain threshold is rather high, I don't mind a little pain, as long as the baby is healthy. Maybe it's because I had a vaginal delivery with epidural anesthesia that I'm so relaxed about it, and I recommend that method to every expectant mother who wants to experience each moment of the delivery without suffering too much pain. You can experience that magical moment fully without feeling any pain.

Some are worried about epidural anesthesia. I recommend you talk to your doctor about it, when you understand the method, you will see there's nothing to worry about. Of course, it depends on the hospital's conditions. I've heard that epidural anesthesia is not available everywhere in Turkey. I can remember the first 10 to 15 minutes of labor pain, before the epidural kicked in, even that short period of pain had exhausted me. The cervix has to dilate 3 inches and a half for vaginal delivery, and the time it takes varies from woman to woman, ranging from as little as 2 hours to as long as 36... Just imagine being in pain for 36 hours – well, I can't. Maybe the reason some women prefer delivering via C-section is that they are scared of labor pain, they think it's best to be unconscious while it all happens and to wake up to hold their baby.

What worries me the most is the moment when the baby will be born. Thanks to ultrasounds, we see the baby on the screen, but it's another thing to see him in flesh and blood! Has he developed fully, does he have ten little toes and ten little fingers? Those are the questions that preoccupy me most during the last days of my pregnancy, rather than delivery, as it was the case with my last pregnancy as well. But when they placed my baby on my chest, as soon as he was born and the umbilical cord was cut, all covered in gooey amniotic fluid, when I held him, then all my worries dissolved away and I was elated.

As the end draws nearer, I'm filled with anticipation. Is he going to be dark or fair? Who is he going to take after? How tall, how big is he going to be? Is he going to be calm or mischievous, a sleepy head like his father or alert like his mother? I can visualize him vaguely based on what I saw on the sonogram but I like to picture him better through my imagination. I imagine Submarine Number 2 to be a little clone of Matteo... My doctor also comments on his appearance during every sonogram: "His head looks like his father's, his facial traits resemble yours, he seems to have a biggish nose. Look, he's glancing at us." When he says he has a lot of hair, Cosimo, who has lost all his hair, beams with joy.

Of course, all of this is only for the fun of it. I don't care about any of this, as long as he is born healthy, it doesn't matter at all whether he has blue or brown eyes, dark or fair hair. I struggled so much to have a baby in the first place that I couldn't so much as imagine to think of such things, my only prayer then was, as it is now, for my baby to be healthy, and when I first held him I thanked God for giving me a healthy baby before I even examined him closely to see what he looked like. I felt like the luckiest woman on earth to have a healthy, happy baby.

Nature Thrown Out of Balance...

It's early September. In three days, we are going to be reunited with daddy who's been away for a whole month. The weather is even nicer than it's been throughout summer, the sea is still as a swimming pool. It's warm and calm. Matteo's playschool is closed for 10 days for maintenance and renovation. The beaches have been deserted since mid-August, as Ramadan has arrived. The warm sea and mild sun are ideal for little children, so my son and I spend our days on the beach. I'm hoping this nice weather will go on after my husband arrives. We hear on the weather forecast that some heavy rain is expected next week but we don't envision a disaster is in store. My husband is arriving on a Saturday afternoon in early September. Matteo, my brother Can, my friend Sibel and I are waiting for him in the airport.

He finally appears at the gate and walks towards us. Matteo is over the moon to see his father, the way he runs to him is a sight for sore eyes. The three of us become one in a tight embrace, with Matteo in the middle, our tears of happiness mingle; daddy is here, even though only for a week. We sit in a café in the airport to start catching up over a cup of coffee, and 'Father Christmas' starts handing out the presents he's brought for us. He knows his son well, he's got him a Formula 1 Ferrari toy car to go into his collection. He's brought me a novel where a mother tells her story, selected book of the year in Italy, besides my favorite perfume and facial cream. He's got Sibel a box of the aromatic teas she likes and Can a cologne. We take leave of Sibel and leave the airport.

On our way back to Tekirdağ, we go out of our routine and choose to take the E5 highway, that a flood will destroy in two days. Rainfall will start that night, and continue unremittingly for two days, bringing a disaster upon Istanbul and Tekirdağ; and we will be watching on TV how the flood washes away the vehicles on this very road to the sea, taking dozens of lives. A mother driving with her two children will survive the loss of one of them in the raging waters. I cannot begin to imagine her pain and trauma, her feelings of guilt, maybe she cannot even rejoice the fact that one of her children has been spared!

The rain never stops throughout the week Cosimo is visiting, and the disaster news don't cease for a moment. Sometimes you feel it's not fair to bring children on this unsound and unbalanced earth. Having a baby is a complicated decision, if you decide not to, then you can't continue your lineage, you feel like you're moving against nature and your mothering instinct, whereas if you decide to go ahead and have a baby, you can't stop thinking what right you have to bring another individual on this unstable planet and feeling guilty. You don't know what to think!

Little Joys

It's the 23rd September, 2009, a big day that will go in my son Matteo's journal. Today he's gone potty for the first time, and we're all very happy. I know it's strange, but there you go, all the family is happy for this. It was the last day of Ramadan Holiday yesterday, but the festive spirit still lingers in our house because Matteo can now use the bathroom to poop! He learned to pee in the toilet a month ago and we haven't had any accidents since then, but we've had to wait until today for the poop part.

I always have a few toys tucked away in the house for special occasions, I give him a fire engine to reward his potty success. He's so happy, he screams with joy. He's been wanting to be a firefighter for some time, this toy engine gets him all worked up. If someone told me a few years ago I would be so happy and excited for something like this, I'd laugh. To think I'm happy over kid's poop! But I am happy, every time my son tells me he has to go. Now, you have to admit it, the definition of happiness and pleasure changes when you become a mother. It makes you happy to smell the milky breath of your baby, to hear him burp; it feels better to see him sleep at peace than to sleep yourself...

This is what motherhood's like. Your perspective on life, your priorities, your pleasures change, you can be happy or upset over little things. Happiness is all around us, in the air, in the water, hidden inside little things, and it's up to us to find it and bring it out and show it to our little ones.

C-Section & Women Losing Their Ability to Deliver

I'm on my 34th week. When I visit the doctor for my routine prenatal exam, we discuss delivery at length. I'm accompanied by my father, who's apparently missed seeing his grandson on the sonogram screen. As the delivery draws nearer, my mind is swarming with questions, as if I've never delivered before. It's a different excitement each time, you feel as if you don't know a thing, and you forget what you know. That's the beauty of it, a new baby, a new excitement, everything is brand new!

The baby's lungs keep developing until the 36th week, after which the chance of survival is very high even if the baby was born before term. A baby born after that point in the pregnancy can adapt to life on its own without intensive care since it is fully developed and grown. You can expect contractions to start but it doesn't necessarily signal the onset of labor, it's only a preparation. On the other hand, the fact that the cervix is closed with a cerclage doesn't mean labor cannot start. The sutures need to be removed on the 37th week at the latest, they are not supposed to be left in place until the last moment, as they might block the natural course of labor. Everything is supposed to be allowed to take its natural course. I'm lucky to have found a doctor in Tekirdağ, who understands and reassures me, and resolves my worries with his detailed explanations. I ask him when the baby turns head down, taking the right position for delivery, to which he replies that my baby has already turned into cephalic presentation, with his head downwards, but he's not engaged yet, which means his head has not descended into the pelvic cavity. Engagement, or baby drop as they call it, takes place in the last weeks of pregnancy and signals that labor is near, and once it starts delivery follows rather quickly.

I've decided to deliver in Istanbul. Not that I don't trust the doctors or hospitals in Tekirdağ, but I just feel like it is the best choice. I was born in Istanbul and I wish for my son to be born in a metropolis like Istanbul. But I discuss delivery options and hospitals in Tekirdağ with my doctor anyway, just in case there is an emergency and the baby decides to come early, before I have time to make it to Istanbul. He says delivery via C-section is the common choice in Tekirdağ, as most women prefer it. Normally, C-section is not an option but a medical decision that the doctor should take in case of necessity, either during or before delivery. In Europe, doctors won't deliver you via C-section even if you asked for it, if they foresee vaginal delivery; you don't get to choose, that's the law. It's only in Turkey that you are offered C-section as a delivery option. And Tekirdağ ranks 3rd in Turkey among the provinces with the highest rate of C-section deliveries. The public hospital has decided to take this increase under control and to allow C-sections only if the doctor thinks it medically necessary; so if you are eager to deliver this way you have to go to a private hospital. Dr. Levent speculates that the trend toward Caesarean delivery will gradually diminish women's ability to deliver naturally, until it's eventually lost for good.

I ask him if the doctors cannot convince their patients who wish to deliver that way when there isn't any medical reasons that call for it to try a natural delivery. He says they try to, but it's up to the patient after all, if they're eager to deliver via C-section, then they are able to request it. Expectant women are generally scared of labor and delivery and they wish to be unconscious while it happens, also they want to ensure their baby a delivery free from risks and complications.

I guess the stories of pain and loss during delivery that we've heard from our mothers or other relatives have marked our subconscious. There is a different reason doctors prefer to deliver their patients through C-section, which is the efficiency of this method. You have to wait for hours for vaginal delivery, and doctors usually have a busy schedule, with patients waiting for them. Also there is a traffic problem in cities such as Istanbul. Whereas Caesarean delivery is a surgical operation after all, with a set time and date, so you can make appointments for it as you would for an exam, which makes life easier for everybody. Both patients and doctors are happy with the arrangement. Now, C-section could be an easy choice in my case; if I knew the exact delivery date in advance I wouldn't need to move to Istanbul three weeks in advance, Matteo wouldn't have to stay away from his playschool and his friends, my husband wouldn't need to come to Turkey any earlier than one day before delivery so he could have more time to spend with the baby afterwards. But I'm lucky that I can have a normal delivery, so I prefer to use that opportunity and experience the moment of my son's birth.

Babies do not arrive necessarily on the expected delivery date, they come out when they decide to. Only about 4 percent of deliveries take place on the expected delivery date determined by the doctors. I can't wrap my mind around scheduling the delivery date to fit the parent's or the doctor's business or holiday schedule. Isn't it reducing the magical event of delivery to a mundane operation? Recently, a friend of mine expecting her second baby has told me that she was surprised when her doctor asked her to fix the delivery date and suggested a date and time. She didn't have the opportunity to think about it and took the time he suggested. Her first delivery was also through C-section. "What could I have said?" she complains. "He is the specialist, it's his call, and he's made up his mind!"

My New Phobia: Arrhythmia

I'm in the last month of my pregnancy, after this point, no matter when the baby arrives there is no health risk, as the baby's development is completed in week 36. If that's the case, what does the baby do inside the womb until term? He grows in size and puts on more weight, in other words the little lamb fattens. He wants to spend a little more time in the cozy, safe cocoon of his mother's belly. Physically, I feel heavy as a whale on land, but emotionally I'm lightened as if a burden has been lifted off my shoulders. I want to enjoy myself with my beautiful belly before the baby comes, lounge in cafés, make time to pamper myself, call the people I want to talk to.

But is it possible for me to have quiet time at all while I'm pregnant! Apparently, I cannot rest easy until I see the baby born, safe and sound. There had to be a problem, everything was too good to be true! My doctor in Tekirdağ told me that the umbilical cord was wrapped around the baby's neck during my routine visit last week. I can hardly remember what he said next, as I got stuck on that last sentence. I guess he may have said something like, "It's not all that dangerous unless it's wrapped around the neck three times..."

I was eventually convinced by the doctor that I needn't worry and calmed down. But during my next control, I notice the doctor is taking his time listening to the baby's heartbeat and focusing hard. There must be something wrong, I feel the color drain from my face. When I listen carefully I can hear an occasional leap in the heartbeat. It's called arrhythmia. The doctor says it's nothing serious, the baby's development is normal but has to be monitored. He tells me not to obsess and worry about it, but it's too late, I'm worried. I'm seized by the doubt whether my baby is healthy and I know I cannot shake it off until he's born – and maybe even longer after that!*

Even as a child, I used to be really anxious about health issues. I remember thinking I had a disease and suspecting silly things. How do we believe all our parts are healthy? What about our internal organs, how can we be sure, considering we cannot see them? What if I have appendicitis like my classmate Özlem and it ruptures before we can make it to the hospital? What if I develop a hernia like Ercan, the neighbor's son? No doubt the documentary about human organs that I saw on TV and couldn't get off my mind inflamed my anxiety, but whatever is the reason, it's a fact that I am apprehensive. Add to that the hormone therapies, drugs, operations, miscarriages, and high risk pregnancies that I've had, and here we are. I had serious problems sometimes when I didn't worry as well, for instance when I was pregnant with the twins, I kept telling myself to relax, trying to think everything was fine, that twins were healthy, that all looked well in the sonogram. But it was not true, the amniotic sac had ruptured and my pregnancy ended badly. When I lost the twins, I kept blaming myself for years for not taking my body's messages more seriously.

The Last Month...

My most important job during the last month is to watch the baby's movements, and induce it to move by eating sugary foods or moving around myself, like going up and down a flight of stairs, when he has remained still for too long. If he still doesn't move, it might mean he's under stress and I need to inform the doctor without delay. Of course, there are times where the baby doesn't move for a while, which is normal, as he needs to rest too, but when he eventually starts kicking I let out a sigh of relief.

I'm scared, I can't help it. I keep asking a lot of questions to my doctor, as I know doctors are not given to explaining things of their own free will – the patients will ask and they will answer. I prepare my questions in advance, as they come to my mind, and I ask them during the appointments. I have delivered before and had an episiotomy, too, but I ask about it again anyway. The Americans love to plan their lives, it is they who have come up with the term 'birth plan', which means the expectant mother's list of things she would like to have or avoid during delivery, of course, it's hard to stick to it completely as you cannot foresee all that can happen during delivery. I don't want to prepare a birth plan but I have to find out about how it's going to proceed and what they are going to do to me, as this is going to be my first delivery in Turkey, I'm a concerned and curious expectant mother...

3 Days, 3 Houses, 3 Friends...

Hooray! I have three days to spend in Istanbul and I'm as free as the seagulls in Istanbul. My son is with his grandparents and my husband is in Italy... Not that there's any place I'd rather be than with them, but sometimes you need a break, where you can get away from it all and spend a few days free from care and responsibility. It's only two weeks to term and my doctor has summoned me to come to Istanbul to have my cervical cerclage removed. Once the gate will be opened, the baby is bound to come any minute and I'm not supposed to go back to Tekirdağ... That's how it was with Matteo, he was born three days after the removal of the stitches. Maybe it was pure coincidence, but what if this baby arrives immediately as well? The doctors won't give me any definite answers, so it's best to be on the safe side. They offer to anaesthetize me for the operation but when I was expecting Matteo, they removed the sutures without anesthesia, so I decline. They remove the sutures, all is fine. In an hour, I'm up, energetic and alert. I go out of the clinic with my father, walking on my two feet, and we head for the Bosphorus to have a nice luncheon.

It's a lovely day, almost like summer, and I've been missing Istanbul, so I try to do everything, to see everybody at once in three days, with my huge belly. I'm supposed to stay at home and spend the last days of my pregnancy resting, but I'm bursting with energy, I can't stand still. I talked to three close friends of mine that I want to see, I'll be spending each one of my three days with one of them. I don't remember having had such a good time in years. When you live overseas it's unavoidable that the time you spend with your old friends decreases, and you miss them very much.

I spend the first night with my childhood friend Umut, in the flat where I lived when I was a student. How we've missed having girl talk! When I get up in the morning, I see I've slept till nine, I can't believe it! I don't remember sleeping this late for months, even for years, thanks to my son who wakes me up at seven o'clock at the latest every morning, no matter how late he goes to bed. We laze around in bed for some time, then, as we are planning to go out to have a breakfast of honey and cream at the sweet shop around the corner, and to read the daily newspapers over a cup of coffee in a café along the Bosphorus, Umut sees that the toilet is clogged. So much for fancy plans. It's an old building, which is the norm in the old city, as well as the reason which I almost always encounter problems when I'm in Istanbul. The breakfast with honey and cream is called off. There's nothing to do but call the plumber at once, who comes immediately, examines the toilet earnestly and declares it has to be removed, with the gravity of a surgeon saying "We have to operate!" Now, that's just what I needed! How can I deal with repair works when I cannot see my feet! The plumber is sympathetic, "Don't worry, mam," he says, "I'll do my job neatly and clean up my mess before I go, you won't have to clean up after me." That's convincing. Apparently, I don't have any options anyway. The work goes on for six hours, but at the end I get a toilet that flushes properly.

As the enlarged womb causes increased pressure on the bladder, I have to go to the toilet hourly – such an ordeal! Unfortunately, all my old neighbors have moved away and there is no one I know in the whole building. Each time I have to go, I use the toilet in a different restaurant in the neighborhood, I even have to use old style squatting toilets a few times, which is really hard when you are pregnant! I pity those who don't have an option but use a squat toilet throughout their pregnancy, life used to be really hard in the old days. Eventually, the toilet is removed, the tiles on the floor around it are broken, the plumbing is cleared, and everything is put back in place, repaired and cleaned. As there is fresh concrete on the floor, we're not supposed to use the toilet tonight. Well, I can live with that, I'll be staying at Elif's tonight anyway. Elif is a university friend of mine, we're going to listen to İlhan Erşahin in concert together this evening. After the toilet problem today, music will definitely do me good, it will cleanse my soul – and it will definitely excite the baby...

❦

The İlhan Erşahin concert is part of the Akbank Jazz Festival. Erşahin, who is embarrassed for his Turkish with an American accent, usually doesn't talk much but this time he surprises us and delivers a pretty long speech before the concert and he is as friendly as ever. As soon as the music starts, a dancing party begins inside my belly! The little one beats the rhythm throughout the concert, and I get kicked continually – I've never seen Submarine Number 2 this excited, it's a new experience for both of us. Babies in the womb are used to the sounds coming from the mother's internal organs but I don't quite know how this volume of sound would affect them and I'm a little worried. At least he's exposed to good music before he's even born yet...

I spend my second night in Istanbul at Elif's. The next morning my cell phone keeps ringing, my husband, my brother, Umut, Sibel, my mother and my father call one after another to ask me how I am doing. I reassure them that I didn't over-exert myself the night before and tell them I'm fine, and not alone, and that the baby has not arrived yet. Everybody is utterly excited, waiting for the baby to arrive at any moment, we don't seem to be able to talk of anything else but the baby...

It's late October, but the days are still warm and sunny. I enjoy the warm autumn morning, sipping tea out in the balcony in Elif's apartment, with a lovely view of the Bosphorus. The reflection of the sun rising over the Anatolian side over the sea is a sight for sore eyes. I'm enchanted once more by the beauty of the Bosphorus. Istanbul is a city where you discover a new charm every single day...

On my third day off, I'm with Sibel. I met her quite late in life but we've become close friends quite quickly, she's been one of my best friends for years. We have a quiet day at home, watch a movie on DVD and then eat the lunch she has prepared. We both have a hearty appetite. Sibel says, "It's quite understandable that you eat for two, but what is my excuse? What am I going to do with this belly?" Although she is complaining about it, her stomach is almost flat, but she's making such a big deal of her few extra pounds that you would think she has a larger belly than mine. That's how we women are, we're never happy about our looks and constantly struggle to lose weight.

Tomorrow, my husband will be in Turkey. It's been nice to have some time with my girlfriends but I miss my husband so much. In Italy, fathers can take a parental leave as well, but it's only for one day, the day when the baby is born! I cannot believe it, I thought Italy was more advanced than that. It turns out my husband, who thinks Italy lags behind most European countries, was right. So he has no option but to use his annual leave days.

The doctor estimates the baby's due date to be between the 8th and the 10th of November. It's the last day of October, so I guess he must be packing up to travel earthbound. The ob-gyns have a calendar disk that they rotate to figure your due date based on your last period, but apparently it's only a rough estimation, the baby may come a little earlier or later than that, whenever he or she feels like it.

Burst of Energy on the Eve of Delivery

They say women get struck by a sudden burst of energy towards the end of the pregnancy, it's called nesting instinct. I'm nearing the end of my 39th week, we expect the baby to arrive any time now. But I can't stand still; I keep finding things to do. I clean up my old student house, go through my clothes that remained in the closet since my university years, do the laundry, throw away piles of trash, organize stuff, tidy up and turn the house upside down. And I make a point of roaming all around Istanbul and enjoying my last free days with my husband and son, thinking I'll be homebound for the first few months after the baby's arrival. We try out the city's countless cafés and restaurants and enjoy being back in Istanbul after so many years. We drive all through the city, with my hospital suitcase in the trunk of the car, so we don't stray too far away from the hospital, as we dread the traffic. As the hospital is in Maslak, our favorite spot is İstinye Park mall. I'm not scared of staying on my feet too long any more, as I'm so near term, on the contrary, I walk around heartily so the baby I'm waiting so impatiently for might come sooner.

And Baby Leo Rushes In...

Yes, it's true that we've almost reached term and the baby is about to come, but honestly, I didn't expect him to come in such a hurry. It's Thursday, November 5th, 2009. In the morning, my father comes from Tekirdağ to see us. We expect the baby to be born on the 10th, which makes this the last week of my pregnancy. I'm going to Dr. Aret Kamar's clinic to have an NST, which I hope will be the last test I have to take. Both my father and brother have their birthdays on the 10th of November, if my son happens to come on that day too, we'll get to celebrate three birthdays in a day each year. My father, my husband, my son and I go out after breakfast. I have an appointment at the beauty parlor in the morning, I want to give myself a full prenatal beauty treatment, mostly because I'd like to be pretty and prepared when my baby comes.

I wasn't well prepared to welcome Matteo since he came early. The mother – naturally – looks exhausted after delivery, if, to top it off, you look unkempt too, it's even worse. Sure, we will not be having a photo-shoot to go on the cover of a magazine, but I would like for my children to see their mother looking pretty when they look at their photos in the future. The other reason I want to go to the beauty parlor is that I might be too busy after the baby's arrival to care for myself, I might hardly find the time to take a shower, let alone go to the beauty parlor. So it's a kind of investment to do it today. For instance, I will not have to deal with hair removal (hair grows annoyingly fast when your hormones go wild), manicure or pedicure for some time. So I leave my three men (my father, my husband and my son) in a cousin's office and drive myself to my appointment in the hair salon I used to use when I lived in Istanbul. (I'll be surprised at myself later for driving so far in my pregnancy!)

Serpil the esthetician warns me about the pain before starting, but I take no heed – I've forgotten what an ordeal it is! And it's even more painful if you're pregnant. Serpil tells me she has a client who gave birth on the same day as she had a bikini wax. "I have so many stories to tell I might write a book about it," she says.

When I lived in Istanbul, I used to go to Zen Kuaför across the road from our building in Akatlar, that's where I've met Serpil. She's an exceptional esthetician, who loves her job and does it meticulously. She's so fussy, she won't leave the slightest trace of hair on your body once you fall into her hands. Her eyes are like a magnifying glass. Well, I didn't expect this much pain, my skin is burning, I beg her to abort the mission, but she won't, "We have to finish what we've started," she protests, "we can't leave it unfinished, you cannot go into delivery like this, half-hairy and half-hairless!" Could it be that she has German blood in her veins, I wonder. After the full body wax that takes about 45 minutes, but feels like hours to me, I surrender myself to the caring hands of the hair dresser. That is my favorite part! The ordeal is over, now it's time for pleasure – I love having someone play with my hair...

The Wax that Induces Delivery

When I tell my doctor that the reason behind my water breaking might be the bikini wax I've had a few hours ago, he doesn't seem to take my thesis too seriously, but I sincerely believe that the pain may have triggered the contractions. He says it must be a coincidence, then lectures me for going through with it: "What did you need a bikini wax for? You shouldn't have troubled yourself!" But what does he know? He's a man, after all, he guesses it must hurt, but he has no idea how much! I promise you, a bikini wax hurts as much as labor pain. I have a high pain threshold, the doctor said that too when I refused anesthesia during the removal of the cervical cerclage. (I thought it was unnecessary to be anaesthetized for such a short operation, I knew it would hurt a little but I didn't mind, I could take it, it would only take five minutes after all, whereas with anesthesia you don't feel that well afterwards for a longer time.)

* Pregnant women who have neared or reached term are usually recommended to get engaged in more activity on their feet, such as

taking long walks, visiting museums or exhibitions, or going shopping
in Ikea, to induce the baby to come. Now, I tried and saw that these
methods do not really work; I believe the surest solution, tested and
approved (by me), is a bikini wax, given by Serpil the Esthetician, if
possible!

When I'm done at the hairdresser's, I join my father, Cosimo,
Matteo and my two cousins in the restaurant where they're
having luncheon. I'm the only female at the table, surrounded by
six men, counting the baby in my belly. It's nice to hear them all
pay me compliments, but the loveliest words are those of my son:
"Your hair looks lovely, anne*, you're so pretty." I could hardly be
considered graceful with my enlarged body and huge belly, but I
do feel good with my pretty hairstyle, my manicured hands and
my make-up. In the meantime, I forget I might soon be delivering
and make plans for a barbecue party with my cousins for the
weekend. We finish our lunch and start for our NST appointment
at the doctor's. We're headed to Taksim, Gümüşsuyu. As we're
driving to the IVF center, Matteo falls asleep in the car. We don't
want to wake him up as we knew he would be ill-tempered all day
if we did, so we leave him in the car with my father, who's more
than willing to stay and take a nap with his grandson.

It's time for the NST: that is the non-stress test, where the
contractions and the baby's heartbeat are recorded. My husband
and I wait for a while outside of the room where the test is done.
When the nurses tell me I can go in and I get up, suddenly my
waters break and gush down my legs! I'm dumbfounded and don't
know what to say, I show the nurse my wet jeans clinging to my

* Mommy in Turkish

legs. She is astonished at the sight and is at a loss as to know what to do. Now, it's a rare patient who comes straight to the doctor's office to go onto labor! I wish I could deliver right there, that would be most convenient. They take me hurriedly into the exam room, where the doctor is seeing another patient. He starts by reprimanding the nurses for letting me stay as I am, in my wet clothes.

Then he examines the baby on the sonogram, who is on his way to come. I say, "You see, Doctor, I've come to you instead of calling you." The doctor says everything is fine and tells me not to worry. "Your membranes have ruptured, but it doesn't mean you are going to give birth right away. You go to the hospital now, I'll arrange my appointments and come right away. I'll be sending one of our doctors after you, to keep an eye on you until I get there." I tell him that I deliver rather quickly, as I know from my previous experience, so he has to hurry, as I would like him to be there. He tells me not to worry and sends us on our way.

Fortunately, the traffic is not as heavy as we dreaded, we make it to Maslak from Taksim in under 45 minutes, during which I keep giving directions to my husband who is behind the wheel and calling my family (starting with my mother) and friends to let them know I'm on my way to delivery. Impatient as I am, I'd rather drive myself too! My mother caught the flu last week and postponed her coming to Istanbul in order not to give it to us, thinking the baby wasn't due for another week. She's upset that she's going to miss her second grandson's birth as well. I tell her it's not possible to know the exact date of delivery in advance, as the babies arrive when they feel like it. She takes the first bus to Istanbul to come and see her grandson. My childhood friend

Umut, who's a film maker, has promised me she would film the delivery but apparently she's not going to make it on time either, as she is currently in Bağdat Street, on the Anatolian side, and her camera is in her house at Gümüşsuyu, from where she'll need to come to the hospital in Maslak. She says she wouldn't have left us at all if she'd known it would be today. Sibel's in Levent, so she'll be there; Ebru lives close to the hospital, so she'll be there too.

Dr. Aret told me he hadn't delivered in this hospital yet. Acıbadem Maslak Hospital is a brand new hospital that's opened only six months ago, in fact, it looks more like a five star hotel than a hospital! Sibel meets us at the entrance, she rushed there before us! I'm taken to my room, where I'll be delivering. How comfortable! Unlike a C-section, you don't need a sterile environment for a natural delivery. My son is too impatient to wait for anybody, he wants to come out as soon as possible, but no one understands my situation, as the hospital staff is more familiar with C-sections. It may sound like a joke but the last natural birth that took place in the hospital was 15 days ago.

The Moment of Birth...

Two hours after my water breaks, the nurses think the cervix has not dilated enough to allow delivery, whereas my contractions are getting more frequent and my moaning and groaning is turning into crying and screaming, increasing in volume as time passes. I urge them, in vain, to call the anesthesiologist and give me an epidural but they insist it's too early yet. My son Matteo is only two years and a half, he cannot be expected to understand all this. My dear friend Ebru rescues us by taking Matteo away to her home to play with her son Bora. My cries alarm my husband and my father, who they rush around in agitation, while Sibel is teasing me, saying that even my screaming is gentle and no one will believe I'm in any real pain if I go on like this. But eventually we get to a point where they do believe me. In half an hour, the distance between contractions drops to three to five minutes, the anesthesiologist finally arrives. He tries to locate my vertebrae to insert the epidural needle, while I try and sit still. I don't know why he had to wait that long, when I'm in sitting position I can almost feel my baby's head about to pop out, yes, just there. He's pushing so hard with his head, he's about to be born. I call out to the nurses: "The baby's is coming!"

They finally grasp the gravity of the situation. The epidural needle is in place but it's too late for the drug to kick in, obviously I'll have delivered before it does. The hospital staff didn't expect it to happen so fast, they are caught unprepared. The surrogate doctor from the clinic that Dr. Aret has sent to keep an eye on me until he arrives will have to deliver the baby. It's going to be his first delivery in this hospital, the green surgical gown that he's been given is too small for him and I can hardly suppress my laughter – I'm surprised I can still follow what's going on around me and laugh when I'm in so much pain. My bed is wheeled through the corridors to the delivery room at the speed of a racing car, skidding as we turn corners. I should be giving birth in my own room but there is no time left to make the necessary arrangements. It's such a circus! I remember Cosimo and Sibel running after me. My father has decided he prefers to stay in the room. Thankfully, the baby manages to come out almost unaided and the doctor who can hardly move in the tight surgical gown doesn't have much to do. Everything goes well, it's an easy delivery. My son is born at 17.15, three hours after my water broke, storming in, fast and furious. The baby I've been carrying in my belly for nine months is now lying on my chest, tiny and warm. I give thanks over and over again for experiencing this greatest happiness of all once more...

When the delivery is so quick, the placenta usually breaks apart, but the surrogate doctor is very careful about it, removing the placenta skillfully, and examining the womb at length via sonography. All is fine. It's been an easy yet adventurous delivery. Cosimo says, "I guess the hospital staff will be talking about this delivery for some time." Sibel keeps repeating in awe, "I've seen it all, all of it!" She's very excited and happy to have witnessed a delivery all through, the real thing has affected her more than the scenes we see in TV series where they play doctor. Everything has gone through so quickly and easily that my hairdo and my makeup are perfect, I'm all neat and tidy. "Look at you," Umut says, amazed, "who could tell you're a mother who has just delivered!" She's filming and asking questions one after the other, making a documentary of my son's birth. Her short film will be a huge success among our entourage in Facebook.

The Next Day...

There's a knock on our hospital's room door early in the morning, while my baby son and I are still half asleep. When I expect a nurse to come in, it's Dr. Aret Kamar. He's all awake and alert, he comes in, bringing in his smiling eyes, his soothing voice and his energy. Better late than never, there he is a last, even though he's missed my delivery. As I tell him all the story, our laughter pours out of the room to the corridor outside. He keeps telling me he's never had a patient like me, he compliments and praises me. "Well done, Nur, bravo!" He says he'll have to embrace me despite the swine flu alarm. I have a few technical questions I'd like to ask him but it's hard to talk when we are laughing so hard. "How long is it going to be before bleeding stops?" I ask. He replies, "Well, I don't know what to say, Nur, nothing about you is normal, you are a special case. I could tell you how long it usually takes but it's no good for you, you invalidate all my estimations. And the baby has proven to be a fast one, he was born before anybody could do anything. When I say, "Of course, I would have liked for you to deliver my son, but fortunately all went well and we didn't have any problems. I gave birth easily." He replies, "Doctors make mistakes, too. But you have a healthy baby, that's what counts, the rest is not important!" It's hard to be outside of the norms but it's nice too. And being a mother again is the greatest blessing ever, it's like having a lovely dream while you're awake. It's a beautiful feeling!

D.I.Y. Baby

Leo takes his position, closes his eyes, buries his face onto my left breast and nurses at length, then sinks softly into sleep. He is now deep asleep, he's even snoring mildly. Leo is a D.I.Y. Baby, he does everything on his own. With Matteo, it was us who wanted to have him, we struggled to make it happen, whereas Leo chose to be born by himself. And he's been a baby who wants to do everything by himself since he's been born as well. I haven't had to make any special effort to breastfeed him, he just started nursing on his own. When he nurses, he drifts away from the rest of the world, he covers his face with his arm and isolates himself. When he's about to fall asleep, he starts to stroke his own hair and massage his scalp with his tiny hands; this indicates he's soon going to go to sleep. And he usually touches my breast or my arm with his other hand. And the position he takes when he nurses is a sight for sore eyes, he's a real prince. Then he lulls himself to sleep and goes to sleep unaided.

Those who came to see him when he was born were surprised by his calm and quietness. People would look for him in his room, not suspecting he slept in a corner of the living room. Leo has always been an independent, self-sufficient baby, who can sit in his stroller or chair quietly and look around him, without needing anyone to entertain him. He has that grave and mature disposition that makes many adults look childish in comparison. He's Leo, the fruit of our love.

6

Final Destination Italy

Two babies, two mothers, one grandmother, in Istanbul Atatürk Airport on our way to Venice. Only ten days to go before the New Year. It's a time where everything is new for me, not only the year. First of all, I have a new baby in my life. A new life in a new house, in a new city, in a new country is awaiting me in the approaching and a new year. I used to be thrilled with new experiences when I was a child, and by new beginnings when I was a young girl; I've always been fond of new things, but this much is a bit too much even for me, I may have been caught unprepared.

What happened in my life? Oh, so much! Being a family with two kids has inevitably changed our lifestyle. Matteo the big brother is taking his time to get used to his new sibling, it's normal, he doesn't want to give up his place. His mother is devoting most of her time to the new member of the family now, while she used to be his and only his before. So he's competing with the baby to be the focal point of all attention. When I'm changing the baby, he says he wants a diaper too and thinks it a good idea to wet his pants. When we go out, he refuses to walk and insists on going in the stroller. Sometimes he has temper tantrums or whines for trivial reasons. When we ask him why he's crying he answers:

"I've become a baby." Now, what would you say to him? I've been reading books and listening to experts, but you understand it only when you experience it.

Taking care of a newborn is nothing compared to looking after an older sibling – you realize that only when you have a two and a half year old 'baby' to care for. As the child grows up, your responsibility and the amount of work you have to do increases gradually, alongside the excitement and the fun. He's growing up, he starts to understand everything and ask questions. If he's not satisfied by your answers, he keeps on asking. He won't sleep wherever you lay him anymore, he may react to a new room or a new bed, or a new place you take him to, he can insist on going back home at once. He can feel jealous, he can't stand me to put the baby to sleep, he even reacts to my sleeping in the same bed as his father. He used to sleep through the night ever since he was a few months old but since the baby's arrival he's been waking up every night and coming to our bed, so I have to wake up a few times to feed the baby, plus a few times to comfort Matteo, to lie with him and lull him to sleep.

On top of all that, my husband, whose office has been moved to a new town, has to get up before dawn to go to work, and I, of course, wake up with him as well. Waking up and going back to sleep so many times every night, going back and forth between the nursery and our bed room, is so tiring that I end up all confused, unable to tell the day from the night. But all this unutterable exhaustion astonishingly melts away when I see the smiling faces of my little princes in the morning. Not that I don't feel totally drained in the evening, but it's definitely worth it, I can give all my time, my sleep, my energy, everything to my sons, who are the most valuable assets of my life. After waiting and struggling for years to have a child, now I have not one, but two children, so I cannot complain even a single day. Today, it's so hard to have a healthy baby. I'm very happy and grateful, like any mother, for this greatest blessing of all...

A mother's life is divided into two parts; before and after the child. You change inevitably, you have to be more disciplined, more organized, or you won't be able to deal with it all! I cannot believe how handy I grew and how many things I can do at once. When you have two or more children, both your hands are always full. You nurse the young one while you're putting the older one to sleep, you play with the older one or help him with his homework while the younger one is sleeping. If you get so lucky that they happen to be both asleep at the same time, you try and get things done while you have the opportunity instead of just lying down to rest a bit, even if you're exhausted. You make such good use of the children's nap time that you get a million things done in such a short while, outdoing yourself. You've become Supermom! But, of course, there's a downside to it, you feed them, clean them, change them, bathe them, play with them, then you do the housework and you cook, and in the evening you are totally drained, you have no energy to spare for you husband who demands your attention as much as the children. Now my life is divided among three men, if I add my father and brother to it in the summer, the number goes up to five. As the three big boys too may act childishly from time to time, I spend all my time trying to please these five men. Not that I complain about it: apparently that's my mission. Long live the boys!

And Others...

Paola

41, Italian

That was the summer when we'd just moved to Brussels. We were new in the city and still in the process of familiarizing ourselves with it. We were continuously receiving invitations thanks to my husband's position being connected to the EU parliament and we tried to keep up with them and to participate in as many social activities as we could. I met Paola at the traditional summer party thrown by a mutual friend of ours who was a lawyer working in the European Commission and I took to her at once, we became friends. Paola proved to be a real friend and never left me alone during the difficult times I went through. One night, while we were talking, she said, facetiously, "Some at our age are becoming grandparents, we are way past the age to have children." That remark impressed me deeply. I was then at the same age as my mother was while I studied in the university, she could easily have been a grandmother, so Paola was right, but maybe a little too realistic. Maybe she had strived and struggled, lost heart and given up. It was as if she was saying our days had passed. I wasn't much younger than she was, just by two years. I still believed I could have a baby and kept trying, but Paola had long given up and started to look for other ways to have a child, which she thought she could only do by adopting...

Paola was one of two daughters of a family from Genoa of moderate means. She grew up with loving and caring parents and had a beautiful childhood. Her mother opted to be a stay at home mom, whereas her father worked as a draftsman preparing the technical drawings of factory and industrial plant projects. They worked hard and did everything in their power to give their daughters a good education. The only trouble clouding the family's happiness was the mother's health, which deteriorated while she was pregnant with Paola and grew even worse with her second pregnancy. She had varicose veins... She had countless surgeries after delivery, developed kidney problems and lost one kidney, and had to wear compression stockings for the rest of her life. Seeing how much trouble pregnancy and delivery can cause deeply affected and scared Paola, but this only lasted until adolescence, where she realized how happy their mother was to have her and her sister and started to feel she'd want to have children in the future.

Paola experienced a lot of parental pressure during her teenage years and couldn't enjoy her youth to the full. It wasn't easy for the parents to have two teenage daughters, both of them attractive girls, they wanted, quite naturally, to protect them and keep them safe, and believed pressure was the way to do it. Paola wasn't able to enjoy her teenage years freely. She started university in Italy but dropped out and left home and moved overseas to work at the age of 20. She wanted to prove that she could manage on her own. She adapted quickly to her new life, she was now a young woman who both worked and earned her living, and had a very active social life. She was very popular, and soon had a boyfriend, a serious relationship, for the first time. She was surprised that her family, who wouldn't let her stray so far as 100 yards from home didn't react badly to her moving to the Netherlands and she appreciated their tolerance in that matter. The years she spent in the Netherlands changed her personality; she became a popular, outgoing girl while she used to be a shy girl who found it difficult to express herself and who was invisible to boys.

Eventually, she met a few boys and had fleeting relationships, until the day she met Alberto to whom she became passionately attached. She found herself wanting to have a child for the first time but their relationship was tiresome; her unfaithful boyfriend didn't bring her peace but anxiety. Their stormy relationship lasted two years on and off, at the end of which Paola decided she couldn't handle it any longer and left. Three years later, she met Michel, a diplomat who changed countries every three or four years. Michel fell in love with beautiful Paola, whom he saw at a party while he was working in the Italian Consulate in the Netherlands. He thought to himself it was the woman of his dreams, which he confessed to her later, after they started dating.

On the other hand, Paola didn't feel the same for Michel when they first met. She wasn't physically attracted to him at first but she enjoyed spending time with him. Comparing him to her ex-boyfriend, she decided to leave him, which was a mistake. She started seeing a Dutch man, but Michel's memory haunted her and she regretted having ended their relationship for a trivial reason, so she called him. They decided to give it another go and never split up since then. They had to manage their relationship mostly over long distances until they got married. Paola accepted a job offer in Alicante, Spain, after a six-year adventure in the Netherlands, and that was just about then that she met Michel.

Her preparations for her new job and new country didn't get in the way of their love. Michel stayed in the Netherlands while Paola moved to Spain and started her new job. After two years and a half of a long distance relationship, Michel proposed. He used to go to Alicante on weekends to see Paola, and one day he showed up with a ring and proposed on the terrace of the house by the seaside, a romantic summer night. Paola said yes without any hesitation. They got married with a little wedding ceremony on a warm June day in Genoa, Italy, Paola's hometown.

Meanwhile, Michel was appointed to Ireland. They spent the first two years of their married life trying to be together as much as they could on trips and weekends, first between the Netherlands and Spain, then between Spain and Ireland. They did have a few weekends where they argued and parted without even so much as a goodbye kiss, besides romantic weekends at the end of which they found it hard to part from one another. They managed to overcome the troubles of a long distance marriage for two years with ups and downs, at the end of which Paola decided she'd had enough of it and took an unpaid leave of absence to move in with Michel in Ireland. Meanwhile she resolved that she wanted to finish her university studies and went back to the University in Genoa, Italy, where she'd suspended her studies years ago.

She started to go back to Italy every two months to take her exams while she was living in Ireland. She spent her days studying, trying delicious new recipes in the kitchen, and exercising a lot. She and her husband enjoyed life to the fullest together, which left them little time to think of anything else. Their life was so full with Paola's studies, her husband's diplomatic and social duties, trips between Italy and Ireland that they never found the opportunity to have a baby, even though they wanted build a family. "We didn't have room for a baby in our life yet. We thought we would get round to it when the time came, we were young, we had plenty of time ahead of us." Paola, who liked a well-planned life, believed she had things to accomplish before having a baby, her priority was to get her degree. She enjoyed her journeys with her husband, she didn't feel ready to have a baby during the three years they spent in Dublin.

Rome... Dolce Vita?

A lovely episode of Paola's life comes to an end with the appointment of Michel to Rome and their moving to Italy. Although they are back to their homeland and close to their families, they are not too happy about it, as the income of a diplomat decreases when he's back to his country and their living standards change. Paola, who's always had aspirations in her life, finds herself deprived of a goal or an occupation for the first time. She starts to wake up joyless in the morning, to have crying fits, and to lose interest in daily activities. This goes on for two months, at the end of which she decides she's had enough of it and finds herself a job without delay. She starts to teach English in a language school both to keep herself busy and to contribute to the family budget. Michel, working in the Ministry of Foreign Affairs, hears that a position as an assistant is available, and Paola is able to get the job in 2003, thanks to her speaking a foreign language. They decide to put off their plans to have a baby for a little longer, this time because of financial concerns, not realizing they are running late for some things. After a while, they decide to try and and have a baby as

Michel's assignment in Rome is soon to be over and he's to be appointed somewhere else, so Paola stops using birth control pills she's been using for years and starts dreaming of the day where she'll conceive.

Brussels And A Tough Episode...

In 2004, Michel hears of a position available in Brussels and applies, with Paola's approval, who doesn't want to stay on in Rome. Career oriented as she is, she's elated that they'll be going to Brussels, as there are a lot of suitable jobs there for her with her qualifications, such as EC positions... She applies at once, and gets a job, outdoing hundreds, or even thousands of other applicants. The financial difficulties they experienced when they lived in Rome are over, they decide to buy a house in Brussels since they like it there. Everything is going well and now they're ready for a baby that they are waiting for impatiently.

But something is wrong. Paola has been trying to conceive for over a year to no avail. They decide to turn to the infertility department of the most renowned university hospital in Brussels, or even in Europe. Several tests are done, revealing no problems, everything looks fine. As Paola is 36 and Michel 43, the doctors recommend that they take up IVF treatment at once. Paola experiences feelings of fear and panic. The treatment scares her in a way she can't explain, she doesn't dare to start. She goes to see her ob-gyn three times in a row, to talk for hours on end. She asks hundreds of questions, knowing most of them are stupid and pointless, but she still can't make up her mind. She's heard stories about how IVF treatment creates changes in the body due to the high level of hormones administered, she's witnessed her friends' experiences, besides the pregnancy problems her mother suffered. All this put her off and she suspends the decision for a while, thinking things might change in the future or that she might come around.

Is Ivf Easier?

Time passes, but Paola is still not convinced about IVF. She worries that the treatment might hurt her or the baby. Meanwhile, she and her husband come across several couples who have adopted and hear nothing but nice experiences, so they start to embrace this as an option, Paola even comes to think of it as the best option for her. She finds the idea of taking a child who needs a home and a family, raising him, and giving him a good life exciting, she never feels awkward about raising somebody else's baby. Therefore, Paola and Michel decide to adopt. They start preparing for adoption, earnestly as they would prepare for an important exam. They prepare all the paperwork. They take a course, several psychologists and experts visit them at home, asking interminable questions, as if they were trying to deter them... At a certain point, Paola is tempted once more to try IVF and goes to a different infertility center to talk to the doctor. A few days after she's visited the hospital and declared she wants to start treatment, she receives a file with documents about the treatment and instructions for them to follow, which Paola reads over and over again, and decides once more that it's definitely not for her, so she tears each and every page and tosses them into the dustbin... without the slightest regret, with relief, even...

There is now but one way for Paola and Michel to have a child it seems, adoption...*†

A year after we talked about all this we hear that Paola is pregnant. It's incredible, but true. Paola conceives when she least expects it, after having longed for a baby for years. She gives birth to a cherub of almost 9 pounds on 27th October, 2010. They name him Luca and Paola miraculously becomes a mother at the age of 42.

----

* It's March, in 2010. The phone rings. It's Paola! Hearing her voice always makes me happy. She skips the small talk, inquiring only after the boys. "Nur, I have good news," she says with an excited tone. The first thing that comes to my mind is that she's soon to be allowed to have a baby to adopt after having waited for over two years now. But the news is even better, she's pregnant, it's a miracle. I'm so happy for her, I burst into tears! Paola prayed so much, waited so much, she definitely deserves it, like every woman who wants to have a baby. I ask about her husband Michel. "He must be ecstatic!" I say. She answers that Michel is indeed very happy about the baby, but there is something else that is upsetting him: They've recently heard that Michel's father has gastric cancer, so it's a difficult time for him. His parents are to come to Brussels from Italy for the treatment, to stay with them. She says, "Not that I'm not worried about the chemo and all the treatments, I feel for him, but there's nothing I can do. I have to think of myself, or rather of the baby I'm carrying right now. The chemotherapy may be harmful for a pregnant woman, so I will not be accompanying them to the hospital." I express my best wishes for her, the baby, and the grandfather, and hang up. This is the best news I've had lately! It's lovely to talk to an old friend, albeit over the phone, and share her happiness, it made my day. In fact, it is babies who make the world a beautiful place.

† I saw Luca, Paola's baby, on Skype for the first time on 9th January, 2011. We were both almost in tears. We were so emotional we didn't know what to say for a while. I was happy just to watch 2 and a half month old Luca quietly. He was a healthy, beautiful baby and he looked at the camera. I thought that was the very meaning of happiness and everything else was futile... Paola was tired because she wasn't getting much sleep but she was so thrilled to have her baby! When I asked her how she felt, she answered, "My love for Luca is so great it's indescribable!"

Maria Cristina

43, Italian

A lovely summer evening in Brussels, Paola and Michel invited us to join them after work at the tennis club to which they belonged. We meant to take up playing tennis again after a long break and Paola wanted to introduce me to a friend of hers she thought I'd like. When I first met Maria Cristina, she struck me as a beautiful tennis player, with her athletic body, her long legs, her white tennis skirt and her racket, although I learned later that she wasn't that good a player. She and her husband Federico joined us for luncheon after taking a shower. Maria Cristina carried herself like a model and sat herself across the table. The purple dress she wore flattered her skin. That night, Maria Cristina, Paola and I had a nice, long conversation, while our husbands talked about games and sports. We had something important in common, which made quite a topic for conversation: All three of us suffered from infertility! We wanted to have babies like crazy but we just couldn't. We were all enthusiastic about sports and exercise and about fashion. This trio definitely had to get together more often. That's how we started to have our 'girls night out' while the husbands stayed at home. I grew fonder of Maria Cristina as I got to know her better. She must have her place in this book with her courage, her strong personality and her colorful life.

Maria Cristina was born in the Renaissance city of Florence in Italy, as the only child of a father who's an engineer and a mother who's a housewife. The bourgeois family has a rather high income level and their life is beautiful. Maria Cristina grows up comfortably, as the only child and the only grandchild of the family. Her parents send her to playschool from the age of three as they don't want her to grow up all alone, where her classmates become her siblings. Maria Cristina likes to dress her Barbie dolls up and talk to them. Even as a young child, she's enthusiastic about fashion and clothes and dressing up. Although she's very active and energetic, she's also a good student. In her teenage years, even though her mother gives her much freedom to allow her to grow up and mature, her father, a man with a Mediterranean spirit, is always protective and possessive towards her. Maria Cristina, while she was all knees and elbows when she was a child, grows up to be a tall, beautiful girl, and she grows confident as she sees how men are interested in her.

She goes to Oxford, UK, for the first summer holiday where she travels alone, at 19 years of age. She has an unforgettable summer in Oxford as she's always wanted to experience college life. She studies foreign languages in university in Rome and then goes back to Florence to get a master's degree in international relations. Although she's devoted to her family and friends, her sense of curiosity compels her to see the world and experience life in foreign countries, and thus begins her London venture. She and two of her close friends go to London to learn English. She makes friends, with whom she travels around UK and practices her English. But after a while she misses Florence and her family and decides to leave London and go back to Italy.

Since she stands out in the crowd wherever she goes, she inevitably comes across celebrities in Italy as well. She meets Alberto Tomba, a world famous Italian skier and they have a relationship that lasts a while. "At 25, I met with one of the most prominent architects in Florence at the opera. We were obviously impressed by each other. We had a great relationship that lasted 4 or 5 years. I was quite arrogant. As a woman, I've always felt superior to men. And that was exactly my attitude towards him. He must have found it attractive, for I felt he was making plans of marrying me, whereas I never meant to marry him. He was not the one for me and I had a lot to do with my life before getting married." Maria Cristina has several relationships, some rather serious, some fleeting, but she never felt ready to get married. "I didn't know what it was that I was looking for in a man but I had no doubt I'd know when I found it. At that stage in my life, I only wanted to be free, to travel, and, of course, to do a lot of sports..."

Maria Cristina has to leave Florence, the fantastic city that she loves, as she finds herself a good job in Milan, and then in Brussels. "A close friend of mine invited me to go and stay with her in Brussels, where she said there was a great job opportunity for me in the EC. I'd always been dreaming of pursuing a career in foreign languages and international relations, it was the ideal job for me, but I had a life and a job that I liked in Italy and life in Brussels didn't have any appeal. I went to Brussels just to see my friend whom I missed, but I met Federico, whom I would later marry, and forgot about everything else and decided to stay there. You should never say never. I used to think I could never live anywhere else than Italy but here I am, living here for eight years. I used to think I could never be with an Italian man, I couldn't trust an Italian man, but I ended up marrying an Italian. I listened to my heart, and I'm glad I did."

Maria Cristina finds Federico very handsome and charming. Federico was working as a war correspondent and he's won the best journalist award in his field at the time. "I was impressed by how intellectual and sophisticated he was." They fell in love at first sight, even though they both have ongoing relationships. Upon Federico's declaration of love, they end their other relationships and Maria Cristina leaves Italy to move in with Federico in Brussels. Everything moves fast. "Federico wanted to have a child right away, as he was worried about waiting too long. But I didn't feel like a having baby without getting married; I was rather conservative on this issue even though I was very open minded on many others." After they live together for five years, they decide to get married, which they do with a ceremony in a magnificent castle in Belgium, and they have a wedding party that summer. Maria Cristina has always wanted to be a mother and she's positive that Federico will make a great father. They feel ready to raise a family. They decide it's the right time to try, as Maria Cristina is 39 and Federico is 35. After trying for a year, they decide to turn to an infertility center without delay. They choose one of the numerous infertility centers in Brussels, but they are not satisfied and decide to change centers, so they go to the AZ-VUB Hospital next. The test results are good, there's apparently nothing wrong with either of them.

They first try artificial insemination, for five times, to no avail. The doctors recommend they try IVF. The first try is a failure, no embryo forms. The second time, an embryo is formed but doesn't survive, Maria Cristina conceives but miscarries. The third time around, six embryos are formed, two of which are transferred to Maria Cristina's womb, but unfortunately this pregnancy ends up in miscarriage again. The infertility center proposes to freeze and store the remaining four embryos, as Maria Cristina has reached the age of 42 by then and the quality of her eggs is bound to deteriorate with time. Women that age are recommended to preserve their eggs or embryos just in case they need them in the future. Maria Cristina is disheartened by the loss of her baby and she wants to take a break, as she's overwhelmed by the treatments. She thinks she might try again later if she finds in herself the courage and energy for it. Her husband respects her decision, they see eye to eye, until Maria Cristina proposes they adopt a baby. Federico opposes this idea at first, as he wants to have and raise his own baby, but Maria Cristina warms to the idea further as she sees how happy the families who have adopted and their children are. She meets many women sharing her predicament, most of whom have already applied to adopt and are waiting for their babies.

It feels really natural to Maria Cristina and she embraces the idea even more as she talks with her friend Paola about it. "So what if I wasn't the biological mother! I was sure I'd love that baby the moment I held it in my arms, there were so many around me who did." Fortunately, it doesn't take long for Federico to come around, in about a year, when he comes home from work one night he says, "Let's get started with the adoption procedure, because I've heard it may take quite a while." Maria Cristina is elated to hear these words from her husband. She calls the same agency where Paola has applied for adoption and the lengthy process starts. Maria Cristina believes it's best to adopt a child from the same race, not because she's not at peace with the idea of raising a baby of a different race but because she thinks it might be tough for the child in the future. She would prefer a European, Western European, or maybe Russian baby, as she thinks most Europeans are racist and worries about the reactions they might face when they go out on the streets with a baby of a different race and fears they might affect her little baby. She thinks Brussels is the perfect place to raise a child although she finds it a little dull and boring.

Maria Cristina and I used to talk about children a lot. Anytime such a topic would come up, I'd always see she was very calm and cool about it. I once asked her what her secret was. "I was disappointed with the failure of the fertility treatments," she said, "but I never felt inadequate because I couldn't have a child. Things like 'You're a real woman only after you have a child' don't bother me at all. You've got to let things run their course, it doesn't make sense to push it! I take each day as it comes, nothing can put me out. Neither I nor my family have a serious problem, so why worry? Que sera sera. There are many kinds of love. As long as I love my husband and he loves me, it's enough for me, life goes on with or without a child. The most important thing for a couple is to have a relationship based on firm ground."

When we had this conversation with Maria Cristina, they were looking for a house with a large yard. The selection criteria for the house were, of course, determined to accommodate the baby who was expected to come join the family soon. Maria Cristina was excited with the idea of becoming a mother. "It doesn't matter how you have a baby," she said, "but how well you raise them... You have to give them a good life, raise them as a good person... I think it's a divine emotion!"

Soon after this, I moved away from Brussels, and Maria Cristina started to have the house they'd just bought remodeled. "A few days after we heard that Paola was pregnant, we received a call from the AZ-VUB Hospital. I would never have believed a phone call could change your life this drastically! The hospital had been keeping the four embryos from our last IVF attempt for a year and they wanted to know what we would like them to do with those. We had to make a decision. I thought it best to donate them, honestly, I didn't have much hope left of having a baby of my own. But my husband was totally against it. He couldn't accept the idea that a baby of ours could come into the world as some other family's child. It was a stressful time. We couldn't make up our minds. We went and talked things over with my doctor, who recommended I give it another go, but I was too scared to try lest I miscarry again. To them it was just a miscarriage but to me it meant everything. The doctor suggested a different method, where the embryos would be allowed to develop in the lab environment for three days before transferring the ones that survive into the womb. Of course, there was a risk that none would survive, but three of them ended up surviving and developing. As a triple pregnancy would be too risky, they transferred two embryos, successfully. I believe a lot depends on the doctor's manual dexterity in this process. I was pregnant, but I didn't really have much faith in the outcome as the first month went by with bleeding and cramps, I lived in constant fear of something going wrong, of losing the babies, which turned my life into a nightmare."*†

------

* As distressful as it was at the beginning, Maria Cristina's pregnancy got better from the second month on. "I think going through all this turned me into a more faithful person. I believed sincerely that I was going to have a baby, I prayed, and finally, it happened. The Lord must have heard my supplication." And Maria Cristina gave birth to her twins, a boy and a girl, in 2011, becoming a mother at 43...

† That lovely summer night at the tennis club, there were three women who shared a

common predicament; they couldn't have babies even though they wanted to. But in five years, the same three women would be sharing the same predicament again, this time because all three had managed to have babies! Maria Cristina receives a call from the adoption agency in the fifth month of her pregnancy, telling her there is a baby they can adopt right away. However the law doesn't allow a pregnant woman to adopt; you can only apply for adoption after your child reaches three years of age. So Maria Cristina had to suspend her desire to adopt a baby for the time being, she would have all the time to think it over as she had three years to go before she could apply again...

Nicole

39, American

Nicole is a friend of mine from Barcelona. We met in an international women's meeting there. We felt close to each other from the beginning as we had a lot in common, we were both married, and childless, and we had very similar life styles. When our husbands hit it off as well we started to see more of each other. We liked to go out for dinner together, to try out delicious Spanish, and especially Catalan dishes. Our husbands, one of them German and the other Italian, who were as knowledgeable on food and wine as to write a book and loved to cook "at their leisure", would be engrossed in "food talk" while we city girls would talk about design, fashion, new trends, furniture, and new venues, clubs, restaurants and the like. We already had having a baby on our agenda, however Nicole and her husband thought it was too early for them yet, as they had been married for just over a year when we met. Nicole was 31 and Marc 34 when they'd got married and they felt they had all the time ahead of them to have a baby.

I, having suffered of irregular periods and hormonal problems in my youth, had two miscarriages, and not succeeded to have a baby no matter how I strived, always thought 'normal' woman never made an issue of having a baby because they could do it whenever they wished, it would never cross their minds that they might not be able to, not a doubt would shadow their future plans. But I was to find out that Nicole had some misgivings about it. When I told her about what I'd been through, she said she thought she'd have problems as well. "My periods have been irregular since my teenage years. Marc and I are not ready to have a baby yet but we will soon be including this into our plans."

Nicole had been in a relationship of six years that almost ended up in marriage before she met Marc. Her American boyfriend kept making plans for the two of them, including all the components of the American dream such as a large house with a yard for barbecue parties, a big car, marriage and children. "He kept making plans for us, but I couldn't see him as the man I'd marry, so I left." Nicole ended her six-year old relationship and never thinks about getting married... until she meets Mr. Right. She falls in love with Marc whom she's met at work.

Marc's parents are German immigrants in America. He is a man enjoying life to the full, who travels a lot, both because his work demands it and because he likes it. He's instantly smitten with that lovely American girl with whom he has a lot in common. At that time, Nicole lives in Washington where she's spent all her life as a child and a student, whereas Marc lives in Barcelona. They have a long-distance relationship for two years, over e-mail messages, Skype and phone calls. When they find virtual dates and rare meetings just don't cut it any longer, they decide it's time to find another solution. Marc, an engineer with German discipline, doesn't feel like wasting any more time or energy, there is no need for them to wait anyway, the only handicap is that they live on different continents. Marc takes the first serious step and proposes in Siena during a trip they take to Italy. Nicole accepts Marc's romantic proposal, which she's been expecting, without any hesitation. Later, the happy couple will immortalize that moment by calling their baby girl Siena after the city where they got engaged.

No Time For A Baby

Nicole, who was a business woman on an upward bound career path, has to pull off the fast lane when she moves to Barcelona and takes a more modest but more tiresome job, as usually happens when couples in long-distance relationships decide to consolidate; compromises are made, often by the woman, who, because of her family building instincts, finds it natural and doesn't regret nor resents it. A woman is always ready to cross out her past and start over, as Nicole does. She leaves her family behind and squeezes her past into a suitcase to fly away to her new life in Barcelona. They have a romantic wedding celebration with their families and friends from all over the world and organize a trip around Barcelona and seaside towns for their guests and have a dreamlike holiday all together.

The couple wake up from their dream to go back to work. Nicole is pleased as she's managed to have her job in the U.S. transferred to Barcelona. Meanwhile, they start looking for an apartment. They find one, in a historical building from the 1800s and remodel it. Their jobs involve frequent business trips, compelling them to defer having a baby. As they travel often, not only for business but also for pleasure, they spend more time in hotel rooms in different countries than at home! Then one day Nicole decides it's time to slow down a little and to have a baby. She conceives in 2005, but sadly, they find the fetal heartbeat has stopped and the fetus is removed at week seven. Nicole is disappointed for a while after the miscarriage but she pulls herself together rather quickly, as she knows many women whose first pregnancies ended in miscarriages, and many of them have conceived right after that and gave birth to healthy babies. Therefore, she decides to try again instead of waiting for the pain to subside, and she soon becomes pregnant again, which she finds out while they are in New York on a trip with Marc. On the plane back to Barcelona, right after take-off, she feels a terrible cramp in the abdomen, followed by heavy bleeding.

As the pilot is debating to go back, they find out there is an ob-gyn on the plane, who has Nicole lie down in the crew's rest area and gives her initial medical intervention. It's a connecting flight to Barcelona via Germany, and they have Nicole hospitalized as soon as they land in Germany, where she has to stay a few days. They find out there is an accumulation of blood in the uterus, which, surprisingly and happily, doesn't hurt the embryo. When she is deemed fit to travel again, she goes home to Barcelona to be followed closely by her own ob-gyn. The test results are fine, but the doctor is cautious, so he prescribes bed rest for the first trimester and rest for the rest of the pregnancy. The delivery takes place following a ten-hour labor and they have a baby girl, Siena. When Siena reaches eighteen months of age, they decide to have another child. "So we tried again in 2007, and in as short as two months' time, I conceived again, but unfortunately it ended with a miscarriage. They said there was no apparent reason to cause it. I got pregnant again in 2008, and we found out the baby's heart had stopped at the sixth week. Each miscarriage depressed me further. The test results were normal but I couldn't be happy about it because each of my pregnancies ended up in miscarriage. I had no problem conceiving, but I couldn't carry the pregnancy beyond the first trimester."

After three miscarriages, two of them in a row, Nicole develops a fear of getting pregnant lest she miscarries again. They suspend their efforts to have another baby for a year, after which Nicole manages to overcome her fear and conceives again in 2009, but spends each and every day of her pregnancy worrying that she might miscarry. As all three of her previous miscarriages took place during the sixth week, they feel they've made it this time when they reach week seven, but unfortunately, they are proven wrong and at the end of the seventh week Nicole is devastated to find out she's lost the baby once more. As always, everything looks normal, driving Nicole crazy! How could she feel like a normal woman after so many miscarriages?!

Secondary Infertility

Recurring miscarriages are common, but secondary infertility, which means failure to conceive again or to carry pregnancy to term after having had a baby once, is also quite common and not to be underestimated. Women suffering from it complain that their predicament is not regarded seriously enough. Nicole happens to be one of them. She loses her baby in her first pregnancy, then she has a successful pregnancy that ends with the birth of their daughter Siena, everything seems to be fine until they want to have a second child.

Yes, secondary infertility is a common problem in our day, of which Nicole's been totally unaware until then. She and her husband are deeply frustrated with their failure in having a second baby and start to resent and blame each other. "Marc is very rational, he's an unmitigated engineer, he thinks that if there's a problem there must be a solution, but not everything in life is that simple and straightforward, and he finds this difficult to grasp. He was unable to comprehend the situation and had a hard time understanding and sympathizing with me. For instance, I'd be crying, and he would say, "Why are you crying? There's got to be a cure for everything, go have a massage or something, relax." He perceived my exhaustion as a physical condition, whereas it was purely psychological. Marc was usually away on a trip when I suffered those painful moments, he was never with me on any of the miscarriages, if he'd seen me at least once go through it, he would have understood, but he hadn't, and he couldn't imagine what I was going through. I was alone when I writhed in cramps the last time I had a miscarriage, my parents were way back home, my husband was on a business trip. A friend of mine helped me get in a cab and we made it to the hospital with difficulty, I thought I was going to die from blood loss. When you are away from you family, your friends become your family instead." It's easy for partners to hurt each other in such a mood, this could easily be the end of your marriage unless you have a strong bond of love and a strong personality. Nicole and Marc go through a difficult time, with fits, tears, resentments, but they are a committed couple and they know they can overcome these difficulties.

The doctors recommend for them to try IVF as their best option after so many miscarriages. They believe it would work because it allows the selection and implantation of the most viable fetuses. Although exhausted from her endless trips to the hospital, Nicole decides to give it one last try, thinking she is that close to having another baby. She's had five pregnancies, only one of which ended with a healthy baby, she feels it's unfair and keeps telling herself that things will turn around this time, that no one can suffer this much pain and trouble. So the treatment starts, with hormones, pills, injections, and finally Nicole's eggs are collected and fertilized. When it's determined that none of the six eggs that have been fertilized are viable, there's not much left to do. It's a great disappointment for Nicole and Marc, who decide it doesn't make sense to keep trying. It is thought there might be a genetic problem with one of them, and they decide to have Marc's sperm tested to see, as it's not possible to test the DNA of the woman's eggs. "It turned out there was something wrong with my husband's sperm's DNA, therefore we were bound to have the same problems if I conceived again; the embryo wouldn't survive and I'd end up losing it.

"The doctors thought it was a miracle that we had a healthy baby as it didn't look possible from a medical point of view. We had to make a decision, we couldn't go on like that. I'd had several miscarriages and felt like a guinea pig. If we wanted another baby, we had to either adopt or resort to using a sperm donor. We thought about and discussed it at length, and came to conclude that it bothered neither of us that I should conceive with someone else's sperm. My husband embraced the idea, and I conceived one more time via artificial insemination and using the sperm from a donor. We are very happy that we made this decision. It was devastating for me to lose four babies. Some couples may find awkward the idea of having a baby with someone else's sperm, but we just wanted a baby and it didn't matter how and from where it came. We are thrilled with our soon-to-be-born daughter. She may be physically only 50 percent ours, but mentally and emotionally she is 100 percent our baby."

Nicole gave birth to a baby daughter in August 2011 and all the family was over the moon. All the pain and trouble, difficulties, worries, fears, and tears were forgotten and dissolved into bliss...*†

---

* When I asked Nicole how she'd chosen the sperm donor, she answered that the law doesn't allow any information to be disclosed about the donors in sperm banks. You fill out a form where you indicate your husband's hair, eye and skin color, and height, and they try to find a matching donor. If you are doing this in Spain, you are not allowed to choose a donor from Spain but you can choose any other country you like. "Our first choice was Italy," Nicole says, "because I am half Italian, and second Germany as Marc's German. Next came North European countries such as Sweden, Norway and Denmark, and the Netherlands, Austria and Switzerland. However the identities and the nationalities of the donors are kept confidential, so we will never know which country our donor was from."

† Little Gabriella, the new arrival to the family, has brought them good luck with Marc's career. He's been appointed to the Middle East and Arabic Division and given more responsibility. However difficult they find it to leave Barcelona they are now preparing to move to Dubai, and they are all excited about it even though they find it sad to leave Barcelona where they first became a family...

Aira

43, Colombian

Aira is a Colombian friend of mine that, like Nicole, I met in Barcelona, in the first meeting of Barcelona Women's Network (BWN) that I've attended. You are usually taken to such meetings by a friend of yours, and it was Cinzia, an Italian friend of mine, who took me. I instantly took to that group of women, the friendliest women I'd met in Barcelona, and I joined the club that same day without any hesitation. I became an active participant in the meetings and activities and met many interesting women who'd come to Barcelona from different countries all over the world.

Aira was one of them. Like many members of the BWN, she and her husband Joe lived in Barcelona because of Joe's position, they'd been living in Switzerland and Italy before. Latin Americans settle in very easily in Barcelona as they speak Spanish. Aira had settled in very well even though it had only been six months since they came. She was a very attractive with her slim, small build, her dark skin and long hair.

Aira was born in Colombia but grew up in the U.S. When she is six, she and her two sisters are devastated by the loss of their mother of breast cancer. About a year later, their father who cannot look after them sends Aira to the U.S. to live with a wealthy family, so she starts to work at a very young age. "I grew up an orphan, my childhood was very difficult. Our father failed us, he didn't want to take the responsibility of me and my sisters. This made me stronger. I stayed with a wealthy American family for five years, looking after their children while I was a child myself. I was swept from one place to another like a dead leaf throughout my childhood and youth, working for several families, which wasn't my choice. But I was an adult now, I could decide on what I wanted to do with my life on my own, I had control over my life."

Aira is 33 when she meets Joe, the man of her life, who is 27 then. They start to live together. In the second year of their relationship, Joe proposes with a ring, on a beach in California. They get married and set sail for adventure. "The man I should marry should convince me first of all that he would make a good father. We didn't want to have a child immediately as soon as we got married. My husband was the eldest of six siblings, he took care of his younger siblings. He didn't like big families and wanted to live with me as a couple for a while longer. I wasn't ready to have a child either, I had to feel totally safe first. I wished for a quiet life but we kept moving often from one country to another because of Joe's work, this lifestyle made me defer having a baby, so I waited for a couple of years. When we moved to Barcelona, I felt it was a great city to have a baby and decided to try before it was too late. I soon conceived without difficulty. Since I was 38, I had to have an amniocentesis test, which I did without the slightest doubt. However, it turned out the fetus had a chromosomal anomaly, it was probably going to be handicapped. So my first pregnancy ended in disappointment."

Like any woman who desires to be a mother, Aira decides to try again. The doctors say she doesn't have a genetic problem. For a year following her first pregnancy, she isn't able to conceive again in spite of her efforts. Meantime, they move from Barcelona to Budapest because of Joe's work. There she goes to a fertility center, where the doctors decide she doesn't have a serious infertility issue. As she has once conceived, they recommend that she try artificial insemination. She tries it three times in a row, without success. In about two years Joe's appointed to a post in the U.S. and they move again. Aira dreams of a baby for five years in her new home in the States, sometimes revolting against her fate which brings her only disappointment when she feels totally ready to have a baby. She turns to an infertility center which has a very high success rate in California to have a go at IVF but this attempt fails as well. She finally gives up any hope of having a baby through infertility treatment. It's an episode of her life where she often asks herself why it's happening to her even though she doesn't deserve it. She covets women pushing strollers, envies expectant women... But she never loses faith, she still believes she's going to have a baby one day and she holds on to this dearly.

Her husband is very supportive throughout this episode. He often repeats that they don't have to have a child to be a family, showing how understanding he is. "It's thanks to him that I kept my spirits high. He left the decision up to me, saying only I had the say over my body."

When they exhaust all treatment options and see that biologically they are never going to have a child, they decide to adopt. "A family helped us with that, telling us that we could adopt from Colombia, since I'm a Colombian citizen. It would be much easier that way. I called my doctor at once, who told me that although he was happy for me I still had time to have a baby myself. I wasn't 40 yet, I knew it wasn't too late to conceive, but I didn't believe it was possible anymore, I wanted to end treatment and look to the future without dwelling on it any longer. So we applied to Colombia for adoption. It took a year to complete the procedure, it was a very difficult and strange time for me. I was scared, very scared. I was under a lot of stress because everything was out of my control, nothing was certain. When was the baby going to come? How old would he/she be? What kind of people were the biological parents? I kept fantasizing about it.

"There were so many formalities to be completed that we had to turn one of our rooms into an office, with a computer, a printer, a photocopier and a fax machine. We had to file papers, fill in forms, sign documents, make payments on end, and everything had to be done by the book, it was almost a full-time job! Each and every document had to be officially approved, we had to get everything stamped, but we managed to get everything done at last and all we had to do was wait. At that stage, it was like we had our hands tied. Everything was proceeding very slowly and stressfully but we had nothing to do but wait."

In Colombia, teenage girls who become mothers and cannot take care of their babies surrender them for adoption. Baby Chloe's mother is a 16 year old student, she's single and wants to continue her studies, so she turns to the state for help. Like any mother, she wishes for her baby to have a family that will give her a happy life. That's how Aira gets the baby that she's been praying for such a long time... Usually, the older the adoptive parents are, the older the child that they are to adopt will be, as it is not desirable for there to be a large age gap between the child and the adoptive mother. Aira applies for adoption at the age of 42, decreasing the odds that she can adopt a young baby, however thanks to her being a housewife and able to stay with the baby full-time, things change in her favor and she's allowed to adopt Chloe, a baby girl only three months old...

A Baby And A Mother With Cancer

The year 2008 is unforgettable for Aira and her family in many aspects. The same year where their little princess Chloe arrives in their family, Aira is diagnosed with breast cancer, the same disease that took her mother when she was a child. Toughened by the loss of her mother and her subsequent life, Aira now fights for her own health. She's brave and calm, and regains her health after a series long and painful tests, cures, operations, and chemotherapy. Both her breasts are removed but she doesn't dwell on it, she's an attractive woman who knows how to take care of herself, so she gets through this difficult time and gets breast implants.

"I've always thought it's for the best that I don't have a biological child. My mother, my aunts, all my female relatives have suffered from breast cancer, like myself. If I had a biological daughter, there's quite a high probability that she'd have it too, which would upset me very much. But our adoptive daughter doesn't have such a risk, as far as we know, and it's a relief. I'm glad I've adopted. I think I've done the right thing. I love my daughter like my own even though we're not genetically connected. She's definitely a part of me, my blood, my life, my dearest daughter! She was only three months old when she came to me, a tiny baby. My husband and his family supported the idea of adoption fully, they were always very sympathetic towards me and never pressured me about having a baby. When I was diagnosed with breast cancer, Chloe wasn't even one year old yet. It's a strange thing to be a mother, you ego just dissolves away; I kept thinking more of her than of myself while I was at the hospital, whether she was being taken good care of, whether she'd been fed, whether she'd slept well... Her existence and my being preoccupied with her helped me overcome the disease more easily. I feel stronger, happier and more at peace than ever. I believe I've been healed by the love and the feeling of responsibility that I have toward my baby."

Gonca

36, Turkish

Gonca is a friend of mine I met in one of the first meetings of the 'Turkish Mothers and Their Babies in Brussels' group. Her son Kerem was the oldest baby in the group, making Gonca a more experienced mother than the rest of us. Kerem is an amiable, well raised child. I've always thought Gonca is a very good mother who has raised her son very well. She's just the type of mother I like, modern, free, and easygoing. It's been three years since we've met and we now live in different countries but we've never lost touch. Gonca's been through a lot during these three years: She was pregnant twice, she moved three times, in three different countries, she started her own business, she failed, she succeeded, failed again, and succeeded again... She got up and went on after each failure. A sunny winter day, she took me to a lake close to where she lived. We took a long walk around the lake with our babies, while she told me her story. She was definitely the epitome of courage, like all the other heroines of this book.

Gonca meets her husband Burak at work, they start dating, then the relationship gets more serious, and they get married in 2002 with a wedding on a hot July night where many things go wrong, they then go on an eventful honeymoon. They go through the first year of their marriage familiarizing themselves with each other and married life. Although they both want children, they put it off for a while as they want to advance their careers and think there's no room in their lives for a baby yet. They take advantage of their childless episode to travel freely, to keep up with their social lives and to enjoy Istanbul nights.

As the first two years and a half of their marriage flies by, Gonca decides it's time to settle down and start to raise a family. She plans to time her pregnancy so she can deliver in spring and raise her young baby in summer, while the weather is nice and warm. Everything goes according to plan and she conceives easily at the age of 30.

After a trouble-free pregnancy, one night during her 38th week, her contractions start and they go to the American Hospital in Nişantaşı. She labors for 9 hours, but the baby doesn't come. Around five o'clock in the morning, Gonca feels she cannot take any more of it and asks for her ob-gyn to be called and for a C-section to be performed. The doctors agree with her. Little Kerem is born in the morning of April 1st, but Gonca cannot hold her son in her arms as she's been dreaming of because the baby has to be taken to an incubator in the NICU as soon as he's born due to respiratory failure. Gonca doesn't get to see her son at all the first day, she is allowed to see him from a distance the second day, and it's only at the end of the interminable third day that she gets to touch and hold her baby, who's all wired up, and only for an hour... "I envied the other mothers who'd just given birth and could hold and breast feed their babies as much as they wished. How natural it looked. While I had to pump my breast milk... I had to leave my baby in the hospital and go home. I was totally miserable. Had I unknowingly done something wrong while I was expecting? I was blaming myself. Yet everything looked alright throughout my pregnancy."

Gonca and Burak go home empty handed, unable to rejoice the birth of their son. They hold on to each other. They're both feeling down, they sit by the crib they've prepared for their baby and weep for hours, praying for him to recover and come home at once.

And The Baby Comes Home!

The baby gets better day by day and finally comes home seven days after birth. Gonca is elated that her son is happy and healthy and sleeping in his crib instead of an incubator after seven interminable nights in the hospital. She's learning to be grateful for what she has.

The first days at home are somewhat difficult. Kerem has got used to the bottle during his stay in the hospital and finds it hard to nurse at first, but Gonca manages to habituate him through patience and perseverance. She's happy that she got rid of the breast pump and can feed her baby directly. It takes Kerem two weeks to learn to nurse. Unfortunately, Gonca has some doubts that shadow those happy days, even though the doctors keep saying there is nothing wrong with the baby and he's perfectly healthy. Her maternal instincts tell her that there is something wrong, when she tells the doctors that one of the baby's eyes looks smaller they dismiss her remarks as groundless worries. But a friend of hers, who's an ophthalmologist, who comes to visit them one day looks at the baby's eyes with a simple light and says it might be serious. Gonca and Burak panic and make an appointment with a renowned professor. Gonca is astonished that none of the doctors in the American Hospital, one of the most reliable hospitals in Istanbul, even in Turkey, where she delivered, noticed the problem with the baby's eyes, especially when he was in the NICU for days, under close scrutiny!

A New Page

"Time seemed to drag while we were waiting in the doctor's exam room. Although I tried to think positively and told myself it couldn't be too serious, all it would take was an eye drop and it would be cured, I couldn't stop shivering with fear." After a few minutes of exam filled with the one-month-old's cries, the doctor declares the problem: The baby's left eye is blind and there is nothing to be done. Gonca hardly hears the rest of what the doctor says.

"Have I done something wrong while I was expecting, doctor? Is it some medicine I might have taken?" The doctor says they cannot know the cause for sure but it cannot have anything to do with the pregnancy, so Gonca shouldn't beat herself up. But he adds that the situation needs to be followed up as it might be due to a genetic condition or a tumor that could progress towards the brain, and could bring about other problems in the future. "I couldn't believe what I was hearing, I couldn't wrap my mind around it. I sobbed my heart out as I listened to the doctor. This couldn't be true, what had my tiny, innocent baby done to deserve this?" How can you not sympathize with her feelings when she's heard the unexpected news? A mother considers her baby above everything else, and would sacrifice anything she has to make sure he is healthy.

They spend days and weeks in exam rooms, hospital corridors, sonography and MR centers, with their baby crying or sleeping in their arms. The results show that the condition is not genetic, nor is it a tumor. Maybe it's as good as a bad situation can be. The baby's overall health is fine except his being blind in one eye. Once more, Gonca is sincerely grateful.

When Kerem's five and a half months old, they have to move to Brussels because of Burak's work. Although she finds it difficult to be on her own with her baby in a country where she doesn't know anyone at first, Gonca really likes Brussels. She makes good friends, who support her in everything so she doesn't miss her family.

It's decided that no intervention should be made until Kerem is eighteen months old. When the left eye becomes noticeably smaller than the right one, the doctors propose to give him a prosthetic eye to remedy the unaesthetic appearance. Little Kerem struggles to get used to the prosthetic eye for six months. He has to stay at the hospital several times for different reasons until he is three, because he's started to bend his head sideways to look, for an unknown reason. "It was like a test of our stamina." Fortunately, they manage to go through it with the help of their friends.

Kerem is now five, a healthy, happy and sociable child, at peace with himself. He has no problem with his prosthetic eye, except having to take it out and clean it from time to time. As he has been used to seeing life from a narrower window since he was born, he's not expected to experience any problems. Gonca is grateful that Kerem is physically and mentally well and happy. "I'm a mother, he's a part of me. Doesn't my heart hurt every time I look into his eyes? Yes, it does! But he is well now, and he is with me, and nothing else matters! We've never treated him as a different child. We've given him all our love and tried to enjoy every moment we've spent together. When we see parents out there worrying because their children won't eat or panicking over a slight fever, we just laugh. They don't know how lucky they are and they are worrying for nothing..."

Kerem Wants To Have A Baby Sister Or Brother

Gonca sees that Kerem is very fond of babies, he wants to cuddle and play with all the babies he comes across, he obviously wants a sibling. Gonca also feels it's a good idea to be a family with two children, so they decide to have another baby, but this time the plan doesn't work! She's been hearing her friends telling about the difficulties they've had trying to conceive, she realizes how much harder it gets to become pregnant as you get older. They have to wait not one, not three, but six months for the good news. Gonca is anxious in their first prenatal visit, but she is relieved to hear the doctor say everything is fine and the baby is well implanted. She tries to think positively, she reassures herself that she's going to have a healthy baby this time...

The eighth week, and the second visit, go by eventless. The visit at the 12th week is considered important. They are at the doctor's office, Gonca is relaxed and she doesn't suspect anything. The doctor keeps moving the sonogram wand at length over her belly, until she becomes fidgety and starts to suspect something is not right from the doctor's facial expression, who finally turns to her and says the baby's neck measurement, 4.2 millimeters, is larger than expected. Gonca is devastated. This is the first time she's had any problems with this pregnancy so far. It's quite serious, the doctors ask for a screening test. The results reveal a risk of down syndrome as high as 1/50. Could a mother take such a risk for her baby and for herself? Gonca feels she can't.

There is a test called amniocentesis where a sample of the amniotic fluid is taken and examined to find out about certain conditions in the baby, but it can only be done at the 16th week and it takes a month for the results to become available, at which point the pregnancy has progressed too far. The doctor suggests another method called chorionic villus sampling (CVS) which allows an earlier diagnosis. In two days, they make an appointment to see a professor who's an expert in the field and the test is performed. CVS is a test where a sample is taken from the placenta, it entails a greater risk than amniocentesis but it's preferred in cases like this as it gives results much earlier. After a long and anxious wait of one week, they get the results, which reveal no chromosomal abnormalities. Gonca is relieved, things look fine for the time being.

The Long Wait...

They have a nice and peaceful two weeks. Then it's time for the 16th week visit. Gonca is excited, she can't wait to see how much her baby has grown. Although she's trying not to worry, she can't help thinking about her past experiences. The doctor says it's good news that there is no chromosomal abnormalities, but warns them that a larger than normal neck measurement might indicate other organ-related problems that cannot be observed any earlier than the 18th week, which fills Gonca's heart with terror and dissolve her excitement into gloom. She's tired of all these emotional ups and downs that make it impossible for her to enjoy her pregnancy. Meanwhile, she has quite a visible bump now, letting her son see that he's going to have a sibling. Kerem is very happy with the prospect of being a big brother, he kisses his baby sister goodnight every night.

They all believed everything would be great and always thought positively. They even decide on a name for their baby girl. Gonca goes to her much apprehended 18th week visit making a conscious effort not to worry. The doctor examines the baby at length, for nearly an hour, at the end of which he turns to Gonca and says that the thickness of the neck has still not changed. "I can also see fluid accumulation around the lungs," he goes on, "there is a whiteness at the lower part of the body that shouldn't be there, the placenta is too thick and the blood flow to the brain is higher than expected.

"The doctor matter-of-factly broke the bad news. We spent years in hospitals and doctor's offices because of our son's health problems, who had to stay at the hospital continually instead of playing. We couldn't face the same experience or worse for another baby. We consulted a second doctor, then a third, but they all observed the same abnormalities and none of them could say anything as to the cause, so they couldn't offer any treatment options. Meanwhile, further tests and interventions continued, fluid samples were taken from my belly, my baby girl was anaesthetized to extract the fluid accumulating around her lungs; her suffering had started before she was even born. My husband and I sat down and talked it out. We had to admit that it would be unfair to bring this baby into the world. We were compelled to decide to end the pregnancy... The odds that the baby would be healthy were 50 percent. Which meant she would be unhealthy with a probability of 50 percent. We let the doctor know of our decision. But there were legal steps to be taken. A committee approval was required for the abortion. As we waited for the approval, that took almost a month, my baby girl's kicks were getting stronger and more frequent every day, making it harder for me to end my pregnancy as the bond between us grew stronger and my son grew more used to the idea that he was soon going to have a sister. The wait grew into an ordeal. As my belly was getting larger, my pain was getting torturous."

Toward The End...

"Finally, we heard from the hospital: The committee had not approved! I couldn't believe it, the decision was like a bad joke, considering the medical facts. In my opinion, it was unfair to bring an unhealthy baby into the world, for the baby herself first of all, and then for her parents and siblings. As it was a Catholic hospital, the committee decision was affected by religious factors. Our doctor recommended we try the AZ-VUB Hospital, which accommodated all faiths. There, they agreed with us and the committee approved of terminating the pregnancy. I had an induced delivery on the 23rd week of my pregnancy and said goodbye to my baby... The genetic experts who performed the first exams saw that the baby had yet another condition, a cleft palate, which couldn't be seen on the sonogram. When I heard that, I was convinced that I'd done the right thing. It was painful that the kicking in my belly had stopped after 23 difficult weeks, but

I consoled myself, thinking I had spent every single day of my pregnancy struggling with anxiety.

"Kerem was too young yet to make sense of the loss of his sister, we told him she'd decided not to come and he accepted it without questioning. The genetic exam of the baby is still going on in Brussels as I'm telling about it all. I've come to Turkey to try and leave this painful event behind. Would I think of having another baby in the future? It's too soon for me to know the answer. It's apparently not as easy as I thought to bring a healthy baby into the world. All mothers who have healthy children, hold on to them and enjoy every moment you get to spend with them!

"The stressful days somehow went by... Time, as always, has healed our wounds, our tense faces have softened, our frowns dissolved, we've started to smile again. We've built a new life in Turkey, with exciting developments on both the business and family fronts. Our little son has grown up, he's now a big boy, 4 year and a half years old. A little while ago, he started to ask the same old question again: 'İnci, Emre and Yağız all have baby brothers and sisters, why don't I have one?' He kept asking for a sibling continually. The subject that we'd been avoiding for a long time came up once more and we decided to have another go at giving our beloved son a sibling. I had no trouble conceiving. But after all that I've been through, I couldn't help worrying about the baby being unhealthy.

"The question haunted me: Is the baby going to be alright this time? The stressful days were back. Time dragged. I went to each doctor's visit with teary eyes, filled with the fear of losing the baby. I tried to think positively but it was hard. The double test results (the first important screening test) were good, all seemed to be going well. When the doctor told us we were going to have another son, I felt the long-lost excitement and hope shine through my anxiety. I had faith, all was going to go well, I was going to have a healthy baby, we were going to be a family of four and our joy and happiness would be doubled. It was time to give the good news to Kerem. When we told him, he beamed with joy, he hugged my belly and started to kiss and talk to his baby brother. He even picked a name for him: Berk. His excitement made me even happier, yet I couldn't help feeling scared. I prayed to God every night not to let my son be disappointed again. Now I'm in the last month of my pregnancy. Very soon, in March 2011, our son Berk will be joining our family. I'm grateful that I'll experience that bliss once again."

Gonca gave birth to a "live baby boy of 20 inches and 8.8 pounds", as it reads on his birth certificate, on 11th March, 2011. This time, she was lucky enough to be able to hold her baby boy as soon as he was born, like many other mothers. And when she witnessed Kerem's joy at the moment where he met his baby brother for the first time she burst into tears. She, her husband Burak and their two sons cuddled up in a tight embrace. Gonca's dreams had come true, she finally had the family that she'd always dreamed of.

Elena

37, Spanish

I met Elena at a friend's birthday party, where she'd come with her baby. I'd noticed that she'd managed to breast feed her baby and lull him to sleep in a corner at the crowded party. Her son, who looked like the epitome of health with his rounded cheeks, his pink complexion and his happy face, either slept or smiled throughout the party, where everyone wanted to hold him for a while. He didn't make a sound, he just looked around, calmly. Elena was as calm and amiable as her baby. I have a special affinity for Spanish people as I lived in Spain for a few years. Elena had caught my attention with her being Spanish to start with, and then with her kind attitude and her placid way of caring for her child. When she told me that she also had two daughters, four and six years old, my admiration doubled. She said it would even be better if she had four children, but three were enough. 'What courage!' I thought. Having three children, when I could hardly cope with one! I congratulated her for having such a lovely baby and we decided we would meet again.

A few weeks later, I received an e-mail message from Stefania, the same friend whose birthday party I'd been to, inviting me to a Spanish-speaking luncheon. The P.S. read, "The food will be Italian, the chat in Spanish." Stefania had lived in Spain for a while like I did and loved the Spanish language. We had a group of 10 women, most of them Spanish or Latin American, where we practiced our Spanish skills. That's where I met Elena again. She was sitting across me with her baby son Hugo in her lap, with all the beauty of motherhood. We had a great time together with our little group of Spanish speaking women who had moved to Brussels for various reasons, talking about life in Brussels, kids, work, career, traveling, our home countries, and food; and we decided to make the Spanish-speaking luncheons a regular thing.

We were invited to our friend Patricia's for our next meeting. Patricia was from Madrid and she'd made tortilla Española, which we devoured with a good appetite before starting to sip our coffees and talk about our stories of labor and delivery. It was Elena's turn. I'd heard from Stefania that she'd lost a baby but hearing her story from her in person was overwhelming. We were all frozen in place. This happy, serene mother had suffered so much in the past. I had to fight back the tears that swell in my eyes as Elena's sad story reminded me of what I'd been through. Her first baby had died of a rare disease at the age of one. She'd experienced the greatest pain a mother could ever experience.

Elena was born in Bilbao, where the world famous Guggenheim Museum is. Her family came from a town near Bilbao where a summer festival was held every year. All the town's people would meet outside in the streets and celebrate. Elena met Carlos, the young man who was going to be her future husband, in the summer festival when she was only 17. It was love at first sight. Their summer love didn't last long, they parted at the end of the summer, Elena went back to Bilbao and Carlos to Burgos, and they didn't see each other for a whole year. "Technology was not so advanced then, we didn't have any means of communication but the landline telephone."

The next summer, Elena went to all the parties in the hope of coming across him again, which finally happened. They stayed engaged for six years, at the end of which they decided to get married when Elena was 24 years old. Carlos was a few years older than her and was working for NATO. They lived in Burgos during the first years of their marriage. They didn't want to have children straight away. Elena preferred to get her degree in economics first, then she started to work. She didn't want to rush into having a baby before it was time, she wanted to set her married life and working life on track first and make room for the baby in her life. She decided it was time on the fourth year of their marriage and she became pregnant. Although all went well for the first months, the doctor ordered her bed rest after the sixth month onwards as the baby was not gaining weight at the desired rate.

Elena does as she's told and carries her pregnancy to term without trouble. Her daughter Carlota is born on a cold January morning in 2000, in the midst of the Y2K celebrations, a healthy baby weighing 6.6 pounds, contrary to expectations. "We were elated, we had our little daughter. Now we were a real family." Baby Carlota's development is satisfactory for the first few months, but from the fourth month on it stalls. She's not gaining weight. For some reason, she's never hungry, she doesn't want to feed. As the baby is reluctant to nurse, the mother's milk production gradually decreases and then stops.

They decide to take her to a pediatrics hospital to have her condition diagnosed. The tests reveal no apparent reason. Meanwhile, Carlos is appointed to Italy and they move when Carlota is seven months old. As her condition has still not improved, they take her to Gesu Bambino (Baby Jesus), the best children's hospital in Rome, maybe the best in Italy. In depth investigations reveal that the baby's heart is larger than normal. She's admitted to hospital when she's nine months old, to stay for months. They wake up in hope each morning, but the treatment doesn't work, the baby's condition grows worse day by day. "No one could do anything to help, my baby was dying before my eyes! There is nothing worse than helplessness!" They spend months in the famous hospital where many sick babies share a room, in difficult conditions, but they don't care the least, as long as Carlota can be cured. As they pursue drug treatment, the doctors warn the family that the odds that their baby will survive are rather slim. Elena is devastated to hear that. She cannot accept it. She keeps praying by her baby's bed, waiting for a miracle, lost and helpless.

When the doctors tell them they've exhausted all the treatment options available and there's nothing further that can be done, the couple are devastated. They decide to try their chance in Spain, their own country. They take little Carlota to a research hospital in Barcelona around Christmas season. The doctors there manage to stop the enlargement of the heart, giving the family a new hope. But the baby still doesn't recover. The doctors think that there is a problem with the lungs as well, that can only be treated with lung transplant. Meanwhile, a sample is taken from the spinal fluid, the exam of which reveals the real cause of the baby's condition: Her metabolism doesn't work as it should. It's a congenital disease that cannot be cured... The father who continues to work in Rome finds the baby weaker and paler every time he comes to see her in Spain, and but he tries to conceal his grief from his wife.

There is nothing that can be done for little Carlota. Elena, who kept hoping that her baby would eventually get well during their stay at the hospital, has to accept that Carlota is headed for the unavoidable end. She keeps weeping all the time, her tears never dry. She tries to manage with valium. When the doctors declare there's nothing left to do, the exhausted couple decide to take their baby home to Spain. Carlota's tiny body soon gives up and she passes away before her mother's eyes. Elena cannot even cry during those days as she has to console her husband. "My husband was in worse condition than I. Our pain was so deep that it took us both a long time to accept it. We buried our baby, but we couldn't let go of her. It was as if she was still with us."

Their return to their home in Italy is sad. Elena's mother gathers everything in the nursery and donates it all to the church before she comes. Elena cannot bring herself to go in the nursery for some time after she comes home. She cannot believe she can ever overcome her misery.

Elena's and her husband's mourning takes longer than they expected. For a long time, they are reluctant to do anything, life is dull and gloomy... They decide to take a holiday, hoping a change would benefit them. "We went on a skiing holiday in the Spanish mountains to recover. Skiing takes a lot of concentration so it purges your mind of all thoughts. You become one with nature and find repose. Although it takes up a lot of energy it refreshes the mind." The mountain air helps Elena to recompose herself. Having spent the last months in a hospital, waiting on her sick baby, surrounded by medicine, doctors, nurses, IV drips, and blood, she needs to find something to keep herself busy and distract herself, so she takes up an Italian class when they go back home to Rome. Her friends are very sympathetic and supportive, they stay by her side through this difficult period. "Everybody says that time is the best medicine, but I didn't want the time to pass because I felt every day erased my baby's face from my memory a little more as it went by."

For a long time, she doesn't imagine having another baby as she doubts it would be healthy. Yet in time, she overcomes this fear and develops a more positive attitude about it with the help of her husband. Meanwhile they have genetic tests done, revealing, unfortunately, that any baby they should have has a 25 percent risk of having the same disease, which is caused by the body's failure to digest the food it takes in and the resulting toxic effects of the undigested food waste in the system. Elena's husband is the carrier. But both of them have faith and courage, they believe they won't have the same misfortune again and decide to try once more. In spite of her unfortunate previous experience, Elena believes everything will go well and the baby will be healthy this time. She and her husband have had a profound confidence in each other and a very strong bond since the day they first met, which gives them strength to go on.

And Elena conceives again a year after she's lost Carlota. Everything looks normal, the doctor says the baby is growing as it should. Elena has a great pregnancy and gives birth to Sofia in 2002. Unlike Carlota, Sofia is always ravenously hungry and ready to nurse, which delights Elena who keeps feeding her, feeling grateful that her prayers have been answered. Carlota had never been able to walk even though she'd reached one year of age, because of her condition. Elena and Carlos think their second child, Sofia, a happy, healthy baby girl, is a gift from God. Two years later, they have another daughter, Claudia. And five month old

Hugo who sits on Elena's lap right now, a real cherub, comes into the world four years after Claudia was born. Carlos and Elena's dream family is now complete… Of course, little Carlota lives on in their hearts, with her pictures adorning their living room.

When I first met Elena, I perceived her as a strong woman with three children, raising them alone as she's far away from her parents. But when I heard her story, I was in awe of her courage. She was such a special mother. In spite of the odds that she might have another unhealthy baby, she'd believed she couldn't come across anything worse than she already had, and gone for it, and she'd managed to realize her greatest dream in life…

Anna

40, Italian

I met Anna when I was just about to finish my book. Her story impressed me so profoundly that I couldn't help including it. Her struggle to have a child, without ever giving up hope, would be an inspiration to many women wishing to have babies. She was a strong-minded, bold, altruistic woman like all the other heroines of this book.

It was a rare sunny morning in winter... They'd told me the Veneto region in Italy had a long winter, now I could see they were right. It'd been almost a month since we'd moved to Vicenza and we were tired of seeing a leaden sky. As soon as we saw the sun shine, we went outside to a playground nearby. First I saw a sweet little girl on the slide and thought how neatly dressed and pretty she was. Then I saw her mother and thought to myself, 'What a pretty woman, and how put together she is! How does she manage to stay so neat and clean in this muddy playground?' I looked at myself, with my soiled black anorak and my muddy sneakers! The boys were continuously on top of me, climbing on my back or on my lap, now, that must be the difference between boys and girls! Anna and her daughter Ginevra came and took the swing next to us while I was swinging Leo and Matteo, and we started to chat. We saw we had a lot in common and took to one another at once, and we started to see each other almost every day. Like me, Anna had struggled to have a baby for a long time and her daughter was born just when she was about to lose hope. When she told me her remarkable story in full detail, I was amazed to see once more how strong and resilient we women are.

Anna was born in Vicenza in 1970. Her father was a soldier, while her mother worked in their family business established by her own father. She had a good childhood, her mother is always there for her even though she's a working woman. But she loses her the age of 20, a great blow for a young woman. Her mother's funeral changes Anna's perspective on life. She receives her degree at 26 and starts work in the sales department of a large jewelry firm in Vicenza, a city renowned for their gold and jewelry business. She's very successful and in a very short time she's promoted to the head of the Northern and Eastern Europe Sales Division. She has to travel often for business, which she thinks is wonderful as she aspires to travel the world. She's very happy about her job and works heartily, unaware that this busy pace is going to cause problems in her life in the future...

"My husband Giovanni and I were part of the same social circle, I used to see him around when I was with my friends but we had not met in person. When I started to work on my thesis, I saw him at the library almost every day, studying hard. Years later, in 2000, our friendship grew into love and we got married in a year, having known each other for years."

Both Giovanni and Anna love children and want to have a big family. "But we were young, we had all the time in the world we thought. We both had busy working lives and wished to live as a couple for a few years. We both liked to travel and wanted to see the world before having children."

Two years after they got married, in 2004, they decide it's time to have a baby. Anna is disappointed every month when she gets her period. She thinks it's harder than she expected. After trying for a year, they decide it's no good waiting any longer and they consult Anna's ob-gyn in Vicenza, who sends them to an infertility center to have some tests done. Anna is then 35... All the tests are done, the results indicating no problem with either of them, except bacterial growth at the cervix, so Anna needs to be treated for it, with a dose of cortisone as high as the human body can take. She's expected to be able to conceive after the treatment, but it doesn't happen. She changes her doctor. The new doctor finds the cortisone treatment that was administered quite unnecessary, prescribing hormone supplementation instead to facilitate her conceiving, again, with no success.

The natural first step to take in such situations is artificial insemination, as it is the easiest and simplest method. After three failed attempts of artificial insemination, they still keep a positive attitude, not discouraged by failure. "When two people are in love, the wish to build a family comes naturally. Yes, we wanted a family, we were ready to do whatever it took to have a baby. Or rather, I was. I was inclined even to adopt, but my husband didn't feel like it was the right choice for us."

The doctor tells Anna it's too early to give up on treatment and recommends IVF as the next step after AI. They make their first IVF attempt a few months after AI, but unfortunately none of the implanted embryos survive. The Italian law allows no more than three embryos to be formed at one time, it's not allowed even to have more eggs fertilized and frozen to be used later on, which decreases the odds of getting pregnant. No wonder

Italian couples flood in to countries like Spain and Belgium for infertility treatment, there are even couples who go and stay in those countries throughout the treatment...

During this period, Giovanni suffers from panic attacks. All the things going on and their failed IVF attempt have affected him deeply. The second IVF attempt is successful and Anna conceives, but unfortunately the embryo dies at the end of the fourth week. The third attempt results in disaster: one of the embryos implanted survives, the weeks go by, and Anna is excited, wondering if they will finally get there, but on the eighth week they realize that the embryo is developing in one of the fallopian tubes instead of the womb. Anna is hospitalized immediately, it's a serious condition, and the left tube needs to be surgically removed. Anna has not told her father about anything that they've been through so far so he won't worry about her, but she feels she has to say something at that stage, since she's alone in the hospital, about to have an operation. She fears Giovanni might not be able to take it since he's already suffering from panic attacks and thinks it would be better for her father to be there to support her husband.

While she's supposed to have her operation the next morning, she starts bleeding and writhing in agonizing pain that night, so she has to be taken into emergency surgery. She comes out exhausted and frustrated. "I had started with high spirits but I was now losing hope. How was I going to conceive with only one tube when I had failed to with two? It felt like a dream to have a baby..."

Anna is sad and tired... She despairs of ever becoming a mother. But after a while she pulls herself together and decides to give it one last try. She's heard of a professor in Bologna who is known to perform miracles. She and Giovanni go to see him, all excited and hopeful. The professor tells Anna that she has a good chance of success with IVF and says there is a clinic in a spa resort near Vicenza where he goes once a month with his team to treat patients. Anna is convinced. She decides the venue is convenient for her as it is close to where she lives, so their fourth IVF attempt takes place in Padua, Abano, but the clinic turns out to be rather unprofessional and sloppy and Anna finds the treatment she receives is totally inadequate.

"This last time was a real ordeal and I regretted having decided to try for a fourth time." In fact, no embryo is formed this time, and the same things is true for all the other women who undergo treatment at the same time as Anna. Anna decides it makes no sense to insist in trying.

"I thought I'd struggled enough and the treatment didn't work for me. Was I disappointed? I was, but believed there was still an option for me to make my dream of having a child come true; I could always adopt, and the idea excited me."

Her husband Giovanni comes around this time, and they apply to an agency in Trento, specializing in international adoption cases. It's almost impossible to adopt from within Italy anyway. Meanwhile Anna quits her job, thinking the company has been quite the opposite of supportive during this period and her work has worn her out. "If you are a woman, everything in life gets more difficult and more complicated. You feel alone and unsupported. Especially if you are a woman who aspires to have a career. It was most natural that I should wish to have a baby but at my work, they were totally against it."

While they are waiting for the adoption process to come through, Anna takes up baking and decorating cupcakes and cream cakes, she does it as a hobby at first, but she soon makes a name for herself within her circle of friends and starts receiving orders for cakes. She and her husband decide to buy a larger house suitable for a larger family. They move in before the remodeling is completed. Anna feels sickly all the time throughout the move, but attributes it to the fact that she's tired and sleep-deprived because of the remodeling works going on in the house. She also suffers from nausea and stomach pain, and thinks she has a stomach cold, but strangely the sickness goes away when she has a bite to eat. She's not familiar with these symptoms, and she doesn't know what to make of them at first, but then she finds out to her great surprise that she's pregnant! For years, she's tried so many different treatments and spent a fortune to have a baby to no avail, and all of a sudden she's conceived naturally all by herself. She and her husband Giovanni are beyond thrilled and overwhelmed with joy. They are a little worried and scared. Happily, everything goes well throughout her pregnancy. As she wants to know for sure that her baby is healthy as soon as possible, she chooses to have CVS test instead of amniocentesis.

Water Birth

Water birth is not an option available in Italy. However, Anna hears of a midwife in Vicenza, who is renowned for assisting labor using water. The midwife has retired but Anna convinces her to help her delivery. When her contractions start, she calls the midwife, who comes to the house. She has Anna get in the tub filled with warm water up to her neck and has her do some light exercises to make sure her labor will be comfortable both for her and for the baby. She's very knowledgeable about all the stages of labor and takes Anna to the hospital when delivery is near. The delivery is easy and quick. Anna gives birth to their daughter Ginevra through natural delivery and she's able to hold her baby after having waited for it for five long years. Giovanni's panic attacks are over. Anna experiences the happiness of being a mother at the age of 38...

And Some Recommendations...

Miscarrying

Miscarriages during the first trimester are now almost commonplace. I, and many women I know personally or indirectly have had miscarriages. When the topic comes up, every woman has at least one story to tell about it. In spite of the advances in medicine, most miscarriages cannot be prevented, still, it's important that your doctor knows you well and follows your pregnancy closely to prevent an early miscarriage. Doctors usually don't consider the first and second miscarriages as an important issue, they only act after the third one. Although it's necessary to take precautions, if a miscarriage will happen, it will happen. It's a kind of natural selection where the defective embryos are eliminated. Doctors agree that if there is an unhealthy embryo formation, it's best for the baby and the mother that the pregnancy ends in miscarriage, which is nature's sound judgment, of course, it's hard for an expecting mother to see it that way. Having a miscarriage is devastating for the mother.

If the miscarried embryo is found to have no genetic problems, then doctors recommend bed rest in the subsequent pregnancies. The cause of such miscarriages is unknown, therefore the right thing to do is to take all the precautions necessary to be on the safe side. This is where finding the right doctor becomes crucial. Supplements or hormone injections are prescribed against progesterone deficiency which is critical during the first stages of pregnancy. Blood thinning pills or injections are prescribed against blood clots that, again, can be a problem during the first stages. Cervical cerclage is a procedure with a long history that can be used to prevent late miscarriages. If there is a genetic defect there's nothing to prevent it, but the risk of miscarriage can be mitigated by following the doctor's advice.

High-Risk Pregnancies

You are finally pregnant, you're elated. But it may not be possible to relax and enjoy a happy, careless pregnancy until term. I may sound paranoid, but I guess that's what happens when you are sensitive. You cannot imagine what an infection you might catch or a medicine you might take during this period might lead to. You also have to consider the possibility of a disease such as diabetes that runs in the family but you didn't have before manifesting itself during pregnancy, of course, you shouldn't panic or stress or obsess about it. The best thing to do to ensure a healthy pregnancy is to make sure you go to your routine prenatal visits and don't miss even the slightest detail. You can sail through even the toughest, riskiest pregnancies when you take the necessary precautions.

In Turkey, 1,500,000 babies are born every year. Five to ten percent of all pregnancies are considered high-risk, which means every year 75 to 150 thousand women suffer high-risk pregnancies, which need to be watched by a special team as they present health risks both to the mother and the baby. Don't let the numbers scare you, you don't need to worry that you might be among them, yet it wouldn't be sensible to act carelessly and engage in heavy exercise at the early stages of your pregnancy. Undesired consequences may be prevented with a little care.

Regular medical exams are necessary during pregnancy, the most important and most critical period of a woman's life, to ensure it's carried to term safely. However, research studies show that one in three pregnant women do not get any routine medical checkups and tests, which are paramount in determining the possible risks in advance.*

Closely Watched Pregnancies

Advanced maternal age is one of the most common factors leading to a pregnancy to be considered high-risk. As most women wait until they are older to have children, age becomes a major issue. While advanced maternal age used to describe women over 30 becoming pregnant once, it now only includes women over 35.

Besides age, a history of recurrent miscarriages or genetic diseases, exposure to harmful substances or radiation, and health conditions such as diabetes, epilepsy, high blood pressure, thyroid issues, cardiovascular and liver diseases are common factors that cause high-risk pregnancies. Blood incompatibility, multiple pregnancies and fetal abnormalities are also classified as high-risk pregnancy factors and monitored accordingly. Some of the most common problems occurring in pregnancies with advanced maternal age are chromosomal anomalies such as Down syndrome. Since Down syndrome is a serious social health issue, older expecting mothers are recommended to have an amniocentesis test done. I thought I was a rare case, it turns out I was among

---

* As someone who has suffered several miscarriages, I cannot help asking why precautionary measures are not taken straight away from the first pregnancy, instead of waiting until after the second or even third miscarriages. I can't wrap my mind around this. I wish I had found the right doctor in time, I wish the necessary precautions had been taken before I had to suffer those painful experiences.

the 5 to 10 percent considered high-risk pregnancies. The most important risk factor for an expectant mother to be considered at high-risk is advanced age, that is, women nearing the end of their 30s or in their 40s.

A woman may find her daily routine and her life style have changed because of pregnancy and feel awkward, it's natural. Add to that the mood swings due to pregnancy hormones, and everything becomes even more difficult. I've read everything about this that I could lay my hands upon, and I can summarize what I've learned about the probable problems that can arise during pregnancy as follows: The hormonal changes during pregnancy may lead to crying fits and nervous attacks. Depression and anxiety are common. Sustained negative emotions may be experienced. Many marriages suffer setbacks. No matter what the cause of dispute may be, the husbands need to be tolerant and sympathetic, and the expectant women need to learn to keep their temper in check using relaxation techniques. They have to make time for themselves, quit negative thoughts and enjoy their pregnancy, so that they can reduce stress and overcome their problems. It's important to know how to manage stress.

Although the negative thoughts and stress are due to the fluctuating hormone levels, lifestyle, personality traits and environmental factors may either alleviate or aggravate the situation. Especially expectant mothers with high-risk pregnancies, like me, may experience higher stress levels. It's hard to control negative emotions such as anger and resentment, which is why it's important to be surrounded by supportive and sympathetic people during pregnancy. You might think of getting help from a therapist if you need to. The expectant mother may experience feelings of happiness because she's going to have a baby, and feelings of doubt or anxiety because she's not sure whether she's ready to be a mother simultaneously. Her mind is constantly occupied with questions such as "Am I going to be able to take good care of my baby? To raise my baby in good health?" which create an added stress factor. If her husband is supportive, she can share her worries with him and it helps her feel better. To suppress these feelings or defer expressing them might intensify them or lead to emotional outbursts later, after the baby is born, with the addition of exhaustion. Expectant mothers can read about motherhood, baby care, or baby psychology; or get in touch with pediatricians and child psychologists to feel better prepared to look after their babies, so that they can be more confident at the later stages of pregnancy.

It's hard to accept the way pregnancy changes your body. Puffy hands and feet, nausea, growing belly and pounds piling up may be upsetting. It's hard to come to terms with your new body that might never return to its pre-pregnancy shape. But at the same time you are elated that you are soon to be a mother. It's stressful to experience all these positive and negative feelings at the same time and stress might affect the physical and mental development of the baby in the womb. There are research studies showing that high stress levels during pregnancy increase the risk of premature delivery and miscarriage. However, moderate levels of stress have been shown to make the babies more intelligent! It requires great skill to achieve the exact right level! Moderation is key, as with most things in life.

You have to accept that you will be gaining some weight during pregnancy as you have to eat a good diet to supply the necessary nutrients to your baby. Don't even think about going on a diet to stop weight gain. Just cut down the three white devils – white sugar, white flour, and salt – but eat whatever you feel like eating. That's what I've done, I ate whatever I desired in moderation, and I gained hardly over 30 pounds throughout both of my pregnancies. Maintaining your social activities and not confining yourself to your home, and getting regular exercise through activities recommended by your doctor, such as walking or swimming, is also an effective way of reducing stress levels. And the expectant mother has to accept the idea that her spouse can still find her attractive in her new shape.

The concerns about the health of the baby will go on throughout the pregnancy, and it's quite normal up to a certain level. But if you are constantly, or increasingly, worried and it affects you social life, then it might increase your stress levels and harm your pregnancy. In such cases, you should find yourself a distraction to keep your stress levels in check; such as participating in or organizing get-togethers, taking walks while listening to music, or finding a hobby.

Stress Reducing Tips For Pregnant Women

• Share any thoughts or feelings that cause you stress with your doctor to receive advice.

• Accept that you can learn to be a good mother 'on-the-job' and from books, doctors, other mothers and other sources; have faith in yourself.

• Share your feelings, wishes and expectations with your spouse, family and friends to get support and help.

- Eat well, sleep well and get enough rest to keep stress levels in check.
- Set aside some 'me-time' and try to avoid people and things that upset you. Some expectant mothers with certain personality traits may unconsciously create negative/stressful environments for themselves.
- Use relaxation techniques (such as breathing exercises and exercises for resting muscles).
- Do the exercises recommended by your doctor regularly (walk outdoors to get plenty of oxygen).
- Set aside some time alone with your baby during the day and talk to him/her, express your love towards him/her.

Bed Rest

When your doctor decides your pregnancy is at risk, he/she may order you to bed rest for the rest of your pregnancy as a precautionary measure. When I was told I had to stay in bed until term, my first thought was how I was going to fill that time. But then I decided it wasn't so bad to take a break for a while and enjoy my pregnancy. Yes, I was going to be confined and restricted, but it was for a good reason. I was going to be able to hold my baby in 6 months, it wasn't such a long time after all, when you think of all the people who are confined to bed for years because of an illness! The women who have high-risk pregnancies are somewhat different from other expectant mothers. Yes, we are more restricted, we lose more muscle tone as we don't get any exercise, we suffer from back ache for staying in bed all the time, but it's not as if we were sick, we just have to sacrifice more for the sake of our baby. It's only temporary, and it's a great period of time. It does bring difficulties but nothing that cannot be overcome with some positive thinking.

Well, if you have nine months to spend at home, in bed, or maybe even in a hospital, you have to do like Pollyanna and play the 'Glad Game,' because you cannot allow yourself to sulk and stress, as it will be harmful both for you and the baby. Set yourself a goal. Although you have to stay in bed, you don't have to be sluggish, languid, and lazy. There's so much you can do during this period of rest. Just use your imagination and look into your area of interest. It's only natural to feel depressed when you have to give up all activity all of a sudden.

You will have all the time in your hands, it's a great opportunity to take up the hobbies you've been meaning to try! I had bought an IKEA table with legs only on one side that you can pull over the bed or the couch, like the food tray tables they use in hospitals; a similar table allows you to do a lot of things while you're sitting or lying down. If you are interested in art, you can draw or paint on it. If you like working on the computer, or surfing the Internet, you can spend all the time you want searching the net, following world news, reading and writing, you could even create a blog, where you can share your feelings and thoughts with other mothers-to-be. You can take steps to have the papers you've written on an amateur or professional level published in a periodical or a magazine.

If you're a bookworm, you have the luxury of reading for hours on end. Don't let this opportunity pass you by! And there's so many books available on motherhood, pregnancy, and baby care, so you could make use of your time preparing for the days to come... If you are a fan of handicrafts, sewing, embroidery, or knitting, you can make all kinds of garments, toys or bed covers for your baby. You can make use of this opportunity to learn or practice a foreign language; you can hire a tutor who will come and teach you at home if you can afford it, or you do like me and invite a friend over to tea, who speaks the language you want to learn and wants to learn the language you speak; it's great fun and it works, too.

Movie fans, you can buy or rent DVD movies and watch all the movies old and new that you've missed. I had never had the opportunity to watch any Audrey Hepburn movies, and I had to put that right as it wouldn't do live in Brussels, 30 feet from the house where she was born and be a stranger to her work, after all she was a neighbor, even though separated from us in time. I had a friend who collected the DVDs of her movies and I borrowed and watched them all one by one, I was particularly delighted by her gracefulness in Breakfast at Tiffany's and I watched it over and over again. Another good idea would be to keep a pregnancy diary! It's fun to write about your mood, your feelings, your changing body, your communication with your baby, and the baby's development in full detail. You could prepare a photo album to welcome your baby, new technology allows your baby's pictures to be taken while still in the womb!*

* I used to envy the women who had normal pregnancies, but I have to admit that having a high-risk pregnancy did have its own advantages, that I used to the fullest when I had to. I was pampered by everyone around, including my husband, my parents, and my friends. I never had to wait in line, everyone let me pass first in the shops, the airport, or the hospital, smiling gracefully, when I pointed out my condition. The cab drivers obliged to take me wherever I wanted without grumbling even if the distance was too short to justify taking a cab. No

matter what country you are in, people have unlimited sympathy for an expectant woman, especially for one who has another baby with her. The doors just swing open for you wherever you go. It's lovely to feel honored this way, so much so that it made me feel like carrying a pillow on my belly under my shirt for the rest of my life.

The Well Kept Expectant Mother...

I've always liked to see pretty pregnant woman who parade their huge bellies in style. Being neat and tidy and all dolled up all the time is not an easy job when you are pregnant. Your huge body takes up all your energy, your face and ankles are puffed up, you don't fancy putting on make-up and dressing up as you can't visualize yourself as being beautiful. However, you have to make an effort to take care of yourself and your appearance, to pamper yourself in order to keep your spirits high.

I've observed that European women are very free to wear whatever they like during pregnancy whereas Turkish women are very conservative. In Turkey, you can only see top models parade in bikinis on the famous beaches, other than that you could hardly see a pregnant woman in her bikini or even in a tank suit, while the public beaches in Barcelona are filled with expectant mothers in bikinis, basking in the sunshine with their huge bellies, and no one finds it strange. Or you can see them wearing crop tops revealing their bumps. Pregnancy is a special condition and our body adjusts to it by making changes as necessary, and we have to do the same and adjust ourselves.

There is no need to make a big deal of weight gain, it's only temporary. I find it's best to dress as ordinary women do instead of trying to hide our bellies (huge as they may be) under loose T-shirts and XXL dresses that make us look shapeless. You might even prove that pregnant women can be elegant too with low-cut tops, slit skirts, and sexy dresses (especially black ones). Use plenty of accessories, large earrings and a scarf are best to complete a plain black dress. Magic motto: know thyself! Try to choose outfits that enhance your best assets. I saw Donna Karan in an Italian restaurant in New York and I was amazed to see how that plain woman made herself look so alluring. She was wearing a long black blouse showing her shoulders – her favorite body part – and covering up everything else. The bare shoulders caught your eye, making you perceive her as an attractive woman.

Tights or leggings and ballerina flats worn under long tunics make an ideal outfit for pregnant women, if they suit your body shape. Don't hold back from getting the items you like, thinking you'll only be wearing them for a short period of time; with a pair of dressy pants and a pair of jeans with elastic waist bands, a skirt, a woolen maternity dress, and your existing shirts, blouses and tops that you can pair with them, you can keep your elegant look throughout your pregnancy. Just make sure all your garments are comfortable to wear, easy to put on and take off, and made of healthy, natural fabrics. Using a little creativity, you can complete an outfit with different accessories. For instance, a pure cotton scarf, a trendy, quality purse, and a pair of comfortable and elegant shoes. Make sure to choose lace-less, soft and comfortable shoes that are easy to put on, otherwise walking may turn into an ordeal with your swollen feet. Ballerina flats are a good choice for all seasons, you might also like short boots in winter and thong sandals or flip-flops in summer, if your feet are well-groomed. Always choose rubber soles or have your leather-sole shoes fitted with a rubber piece, as leather soles have a poor grip on pavement and tend to slip. Wide black sunglasses are a life saver when your eyes look tired after a sleepless night or when you can't be bothered to put make-up on your weary face. You won't always feel up to dolling yourself up every time you are stepping out of the house, get a beret into which you can tuck your unkempt hair and hide it from view when you have to; it will give you a trendy maternity look, it doesn't hurt to try.

The Sophia Loren Bra

A well-groomed woman has more confidence in herself, she even stands taller, so it's important to make time for self-care and hygiene throughout pregnancy. Take my word for it, you'll feel happier with yourself. Besides, it doesn't make sense to stress about your changing looks and think you're getting ugly, it all depends on how you look at it. Pregnancy makes you look prettier, if anything. It's up to us to bring out that prettiness. You have to see the bright side of getting larger. For instance, your skin will be firmer, your hair and nails will be stronger (probably due the effect of your hormones and the vitamin supplements that you are taking). Your breasts will be fuller and firmer than they've ever been in your life – better breasts without implants, what more could you ask for? Why not get a pretty low-cut shirt and enjoy our new looks? Indulge in Sophia Loren style bras and low-cut blouses to pamper both yourself and your spouse.

While taking good care of your belly during pregnancy, do

not neglect your breast; as they get fuller and heavier the skin will stretch, which might lead to stretch marks. Tenderness, sore nipples and itchiness are common breast complaints in pregnancy. I've had them all at different times. It's easy to take care of your breasts, and it's fun, too. Start with applying cold water to your breasts for a short time before you finish showering, it will enhance blood flow. Then dry yourself up and apply baby oil or vitamin E on your breasts with light, massaging strokes to strengthen collagen tissue. Wipe the breasts with a cloth, rub body lotion all over your body, and you're done! It's best to do it daily if you can, but I wasn't that diligent about it, I usually did it once or twice a week. Well, I guess it's still better than nothing.

Your changing hormone levels and increasing body weight can make it difficult to get out of bed in the morning. If you're having difficulty starting the day, the best solution is, again, taking a shower. You may find it hard to get yourself out of your warm bed and into the shower but it will give you renewed vigor and confidence when you're feeling like an elephant.

Varicose veins are a common complaint during pregnancy. I had them even before pregnancy, and they grew worse when I got pregnant. The growing uterus hinders blood circulation to the heart, causing extra pressure on blood vessels in the legs. To mitigate it, I showered my feet and lower legs with cold water every morning, as recommended by my doctor. Cold water exercises the blood vessels by making them contract. Foot exercises and light massage are also very beneficial. Swimming, walking and passive exercise are also recommended to prevent varicose veins formation during pregnancy.

Our feet carry all the load of our body, which increases

tremendously during pregnancy. I was lucky that I didn't have swelling and pain in my feet, but for those who do, I recommend foot massage or foot exercises. The easiest thing you can do to remedy aching feet is to roll a tennis ball under the ball of your foot or walk bare foot on grass, gravel or sand. These interesting activities are recommended even more when you're pregnant as different textures have a massaging effect on feet and activate the reflex regions in the feet.

Water, plenty of oxygen and sun are the essential elements for a pregnant woman. The sun cheered me up instantly in the mornings where I woke up in low spirits. We all know that the sun increases bone strength but recently we've been worried about the harmful effects of sun rays because of the thinning of the ozone layer. Use sunscreen with a good SPF to enjoy the benefits of sunshine without feeling guilty. Watch out for pigmentation marks. Our skin becomes more sensitive during pregnancy as we produce more pigment, spots and freckles increase, blemishes become more marked. When I was pregnant with my first son, I developed blotches over my body. My skin care specialist told me not to worry and that they should disappear after delivery, which they did, my skin returned to its pre-pregnancy state after delivery. Hair care is also important in as our hair brings out the beauty of our face.

It's a must to get rid of unwanted hair, whether or not we like wearing miniskirts. Even if you have to spend your pregnancy at home, it feels good to have smooth, hairless skin. You can give yourself a full body treatment at home with a fragrant skin care product that will freshen your skin, you will find it feels good to touch yourself, too. I'm against investing a fortune on skin care products. Cucumbers and peaches make excellent natural skin masks. When you peel a cucumber or a peach, apply the skin on your face as a cooling mask, or cut them in slices and apply on your face. I use the fresh cucumbers picked from the greenhouse in our garden, you couldn't get a better product for any amount of money.

Would That Hurt The Baby?

"Would that hurt the baby?" This is one of the most common questions asked by expectant mothers. We are confused by the misleading bits of information that we hear around and the pointless news and articles that appear in the media, what's said to be good for you one day may be declared harmful or carcinogenic the next day. When I come across contradictory bits of information, I ask two or more doctors for their opinion, search the net, and blend all the information I get with my intuition to make a decision.

Dyeing your hair during pregnancy: I wasn't able to get a clear cut answer from anyone so far as to whether dyeing your hair while you're pregnant may cause any harm to the baby. There is no evidence that hair dyeing hurts the baby; even though there are differing opinions, doctors generally agree that the dye is unlikely to reach the baby. However, you are recommended to select natural dyes.

Getting massages: Massages don't hurt the baby. I had a therapeutic massage called kinotherapy, which is similar to physiotherapy, when I was pregnant with Matteo and I was very pleased with the results.

Swimming in the sea: The sea is always safer than a swimming pool and swimming in the sea is totally alright during pregnancy. Just don't sit around in a wet bathing suit; moisture triggers yeast infections.

Exercising: Exercising makes delivery easier. If your doctor approves and you feel up to it, you're lucky, don't hold back.

Pregnancy Doesn't Ruin Your Body!

Most of us are worried about how our bodies will look after delivery and how long it will take us to get back to our pre-pregnancy shape. It's no good worrying about weight gain or stretch marks, our genes determine how our body is affected with pregnancy. I don't want to dishearten you, but if you will get stretch marks, then you will, no matter what cream you rub on your belly. The elasticity of the skin varies from woman to woman. If your mother didn't get them, you're lucky, it improves your odds more than the best cream, you probably won't get any stretch marks either. But it doesn't hurt to take precautions to decrease skin marks. Almond oil – that's been used for ages by pregnant women – is the best solution, it nourishes the skin and it can be used as a massage oil. It's very effective against itchy, irritated skin and stretch marks. I found it comforting to rub cream on my body, I tried to do it regularly, especially on my belly and thighs. It also gave me a feeling of stroking and getting in touch with my baby.

Fluid retention is one of the most common complaints during pregnancy. I was lucky that I didn't suffer from it. Just imagine your feet and ankles swelling while your belly is bulging, how terrible is that! I recommend those who suffer from fluid retention to drink a lot of water, linden and fennel herbal teas, and to eat green vegetables that contain water, especially cucumbers. I am a great fan of fennel tea; although it's not widely used in Turkey, it's highly recommended by doctors, dieticians, pediatric nurses in Europe to be consumed by all, and especially by nursing mothers. The aroma and flavor of fennel may seem too strong at first but you get to like it in time as you get used to it. It also helps against indigestion, heart burn, nausea and flatulence, all common pregnancy complaints. And it's believed to stimulate milk production from the 40th week of pregnancy onwards, so it's recommended for use after delivery, too.

Tough Pregnancies

There are women who sail through pregnancy with just 15 pounds of weight gain. They look more like a little bloated than pregnant, if you saw them from behind, you wouldn't know they are expecting. They never give up exercising, they keep doing whatever they did before getting pregnant and don't change their life style. I wasn't supposed to do any exercise during pregnancy, and I envied the pregnant women who did yoga or pilates, cycled, went to the gym or to the swimming pool. If you have a pregnancy without complications, any exercise that your doctor will approve of is beneficial for you. Let alone light exercises, I've even seen pregnant women go skiing. A friend of mine from Belgium went skiing when she was seven months along, I asked her what her doctor had to say about it, she answered: "He just told me to be careful."

The northern people are so laidback, we Mediterranean

people just can't believe it. Inversely, our emotionality surprises them. Cool expectant women that we might envy walk around in stiletto heels, go to cocktail parties, travel around the world, and sail through pregnancy gracefully. On the other hand, there are those who have to watch every step they take throughout their pregnancy and still can't escape trouble.

My friend Narden from Cyprus is one of them: She had gestational diabetes that manifested itself on the 24th week of her pregnancy. She followed a very strict diet and managed to deliver a healthy baby. She had the same condition again in her second pregnancy, and she managed more easily this time as she was more experienced and calm. Another friend of mine had to deliver through C-section as her blood pressure spiked up during delivery.

My friend Yasmin, who was pregnant with twins, started feeling an awful pain in her left hip on the sixth month. She was diagnosed with avascular necrosis, meaning death of bone tissue due to a lack of blood supply. She had a blood vessel compressed, compromising blood flow, although she hadn't put on excessive weight. Furthermore, there was edema on the same hip. She wasn't supposed to take any drugs since she was pregnant, so she was ordered bed rest for the rest of her pregnancy. But as if that wasn't enough, she had a terrible surprise on the 31st week: The amniotic sac of one of the twins was ruptured. She could go on with her pregnancy like that for only eight days, during which she was put on cortisone to stimulate the babies' lung development. The treatment was effective and saved the twins, but caused further harm to Yasmin's bones. The babies were delivered via C-section at the end of the 31st week and taken into an incubator for a while, after which they were allowed to be taken home. But Yasmin's problem persisted after delivery and she had a tough time taking care of the twins with her aching hip. But after a while her edema cleared up without any medication, and, by walking and sunbathing, she managed to restore the strength of her hip bones again and to go back to her life as usual.

Ebru is a very close friend of mine who had a very difficult pregnancy. She didn't experience any complications the first time she was pregnant, but the second time around, she had to deal with all sorts of problems. She first found out she was expecting twins, but after a while one of the babies died. She had bleeding, which created a high risk of miscarriage, so she was ordered strict bed rest for the first trimester, during which she struggled with nausea and vomiting, and terrible stomach pains.

The gravity of the condition became apparent when she saw blood in her vomit one day. She was diagnosed with ulcer of the stomach, but being pregnant, she couldn't use medicines and she couldn't have an endoscopy, so she just had to put up with the pain. Fortunately, they were able to find a doctor who was an expert in such cases, and put Ebru on a medicine used for advanced cancer patients to heal the wound, which turned out to be effective. If the wound didn't heal, they were going to be compelled to end the pregnancy. Ebru endured the pain, and the need to take endless trips to the bathroom. Seeing his mother suffer like that affected the psychological stability of Bora, her five year old son, who started to fear that his mother was going to die. Ebru says she was so exhausted that she wasn't able to take care of her son, and it made her even more miserable. She didn't want to explain to him that her problems were related to her pregnancy because she thought he might blame his sibling to be born. She did an amniocentesis test both because of her age (she was 36) and because she was worried about the drugs she was taking hurting the baby. Somehow, they had to insert the needle twice, which increased the risk of the sac being ruptured, and Ebru was confined to bed once more. Fortunately, the results were good. But before she could enjoy any relief, the varicose veins in her legs started to worsen; she was having difficulty moving around and suffering from cramps while walking.

She also developed varicose veins in the vulva, as the veins around the vagina were swollen due to pregnancy. She had to be very careful because the swollen veins were susceptible to bleeding. She was also told that she might need a C-section as vaginal delivery could be impossible. She had to wear compression stockings that came up to her groin. As if she didn't have enough problems as it were, her teeth were decaying and she developed gum problems because of the hormonal imbalance and calcium deficiency due to pregnancy. She had to visit the dentist several times to have her swollen gums and decaying teeth looked at, but not much could be done while she was pregnant, except a root canal treatment on two teeth.

Then she went down with the swine flu; her son had carried the virus home from school. She passed out and was hospitalized. She was held in quarantine for three days, with high fever and vomiting. When she returned home from the hospital, she was positive that she'd had more than her share of troubles, but she was wrong. After a while, she started itching all over. At the beginning she thought it was an allergic reaction to something she'd had, and had to see a doctor when the itching wouldn't subside. As she was pregnant, she could not be prescribed any medicine for allergy. But it became so bad that she found herself in the bathtub, scratching her itchy skin with a fork!

When her husband Tamer saw that, he decided to take her to the hospital once more. The tests revealed that her liver enzymes were higher than normal. Her blood and urine had to be tested everyday. When she was through her 32nd week, she experienced serious weight loss and loss of sleep, she felt constantly exhausted. On the 34th week, the doctor decided that her liver was failing and waiting even one more day might result in the loss of the baby and in Ebru going into a coma, so they performed a C-section to deliver the baby. When, miraculously, her baby girl was born healthy after all that, Ebru finally sighed in relief. She says "It was worth all that I'd been through. All the pains and difficulties were forgotten."

All of those were terribly difficult pregnancies. But the worst thing that can happen to a pregnant woman is the onset of contractions early in the pregnancy. The contractions are not supposed to start until the last weeks, if they start to early trough the pregnancy the doctor will keep the mother under close watch and prescribe bed rest. My friend Gloria is one of the women who have experienced that. Her contractions started quite strongly on the sixth month, so she had to spend the last trimester in bed. But she managed to carry her pregnancy to term in spite of the frequent contractions.

Morning Sickness, Day And Night!

The first trimester of pregnancy might be marked by morning sickness. You don't know what to eat, and the best way of quelling nausea is consuming carbohydrates, so you might find yourself feeding on bread or pasta or bread sticks when you're supposed to eat a varied diet during pregnancy. These life-saving carbs may also be full of calories. Some women are so badly affected by morning sickness that they cannot eat at all, some may not even drink water. The hormonal changes in pregnancy increase a woman's sensitivity to smells. I know some expectant women who couldn't go out because they couldn't stand people's smell, and some lost weight because they couldn't eat. Unfortunately, there isn't much you can do about it as it's not recommended that you should use medicines during pregnancy, so you have to wait until the first trimester is over, and sometimes until the end of the fourth month. I didn't suffer too badly from morning sickness, but I couldn't stand the smell of toothpaste, deodorants and coffee, so I had to avoid them for 9 months.

It's Alright To Put On Weight During Pregnancy

Nausea subsides at the end of the third, or at most the fourth month. During the second trimester you will feel more energetic. You will also have a healthy appetite and you will be craving strange things. From the fourth month onward, weight gain will pick up. I was pregnant during the Cherry Festival in Tekirdağ. I'm very fond of fruit, especially of cherries, I'd easily eat two pounds of them at once. You are allowed to eat four or five servings of fruit a day during pregnancy, and a dozen cherries make up one serving. Who could be satisfied by a dozen cherries? Definitely not me! I once counted the cherries I ate at one go, I'd eaten 67, which was more than my total daily allowance of fruit! If I put on too much weight on the fourth month, the culprit was obvious: cherries! It's alright to eat anything during pregnancy but you shouldn't overdo it.

You put on weight, but for a good cause; you have to nourish your baby so it grows and develops. Normally it upsets me when I cannot fit in my clothes, but when you're pregnant you don't mind, you have an excuse! You're expected to gain 20 to 33 pounds but your doctor's expectancy might be somewhat different, mine was very particular about weight gain and I was allowed to gain no more than 26 pounds total. If on a particular appointment, it turned out I'd exceeded the limit for that month, I was in for it: "You've been eating for two, huh?" she'd say. The doctors are not happy about your putting on too much weight when you're nearing delivery, as the extra pounds may complicate things. Contrary to general belief, the baby's weight doesn't increase in proportion to the amount of weight the mother puts on; no matter how many extra pounds you gain, the baby will only be as plump as it needs to be, the rest will be stored in your thighs!

About the foods that you're not supposed to eat during pregnancy, I've come across many different opinions as I've consulted with different doctors in different countries. In Spain, doctors don't mention ham and bacon when they list the foods that are off limits. Spanish women couldn't (or wouldn't) give it up anyway even if it was forbidden, as it is a staple food in Spain, people wouldn't dream of going without it.* On the other hand,

---

* Ham is an important food to the Spanish people. One day after we'd recently moved to Barcelona, my husband and I went out for luncheon, but I had a stomach ache and

in Turkey and Belgium, expectant women are recommended to consume smoked or processed meats like ham or sausages only after cooking thoroughly, if they have to eat them at all. Cheese is another matter of controversy. Especially in Turkey, a real heaven for cheese lovers, be wary of cheeses produced in uncontrolled dairies, as unpasteurized soft cheeses may harbor bacteria, which may be transmitted to the baby through the placenta. Pregnant women in Italy are not advised against consuming Parmesan, while most books about pregnancy written by American experts list it among the types of cheese you're not supposed to consume. Experts in the UK maintain that liver may cause deformations in babies due to its high content of vitamin A, while Turkish doctors recommend it to pregnant women. Sushi is another source of confusion: In most countries it's not recommended as it contains raw fish, but raw fish and sushi are highly common and popular in Japan, where they are produced in very controlled environments. Whereas the jury is still out on some foods, there are certain food items that are considered a no-no by all the experts worldwide, such as blue cheeses, caffeinated beverages, raw eggs, and raw crustaceans/shell fish.

The doctors' opinions also vary about alcoholic beverages. My Sri-Lankan friend Aiasha was recommended to take two glasses of wine a week while she was pregnant with her second child. In Belgium, where beer is very popular, doctors allow one

---

I didn't feel like I was up to eating anything. The chef recommended that I eat a ham sandwich as it was the best thing for an upset stomach. I thought I'd misunderstood him because of my poor Spanish, but it turned out it was exactly what he was saying, and he was not joking, either. Apparently, ham is the cure for all ailments in Spain!

or two small glasses of beer a week, but the doctors I was seeing told me to avoid alcohol, some even said I wasn't supposed to take a single sip, but I thought it alright to drink a little bit of wine or Champagne when we were celebrating something. But I usually tried to avoid the foods I had any doubts about or were not recommended by the doctors; pregnancy is only a temporary situation after all, it lasts but nine months, so it shouldn't be that difficult to go without some foods for the duration. You might think of it as a detox program. Just think of those who have to forgo some food items because of allergies, intolerance, or other diseases for the rest of their lives, and be grateful!*

The Italians are obsessed with hygiene! They have to disinfect absolutely everything. They wash produce in disinfecting solution. They sterilize all the items, the food and drink containers, everything that the baby will use. They use Napisan, a disinfecting solution, besides detergent to wash their clothes. Italian doctors prohibit the consumption of salads anywhere but at home throughout pregnancy, as washing the herbs and other ingredients with water won't do, they have to be washed with a special disinfecting solution to kill the bacteria.

After Delivery

As I spent my pregnancy lying down, my muscles were weakened. Looking after a newborn baby is very enjoyable, but it is hard work. You don't have a minute's break, you have to feed, burp, change, and bathe the baby, besides the usual cleaning, laundry, ironing, and other chores around the house... You have to be in good shape to survive this hectic pace. But my body was not up to it. I found it hard to climb the 10-step stair within the house, my knees hurt! When your muscles are strong, the burden on the joints is not too heavy, but when your muscles are weak, like mine were, the joints suffer from it. I had to find a solution, and I knew what it was: I had to exercise and lose weight. You have to give your body at least six months', or even a year's time to recover after delivery. It's amazing how some models or actresses go back on the catwalk or on the stage in a few months after they've had a baby. I admit that their bodies are their capital assets and they invest a fortune on getting back in shape as soon as possible, but it's still irritating; when you see them on the cover of a magazine, slender as a reed, you wonder where the baby has come from. We ordinary women cannot be expected to spend our whole day accompanied by a personal trainer and a dietician, we cannot afford that. Don't expect miracles in too short a time period even if you follow a diet besides exercising, you'll only make yourself miserable if you push it too hard because it's a time where your hormone levels still fluctuate.

When you step on the scale postpartum, you'll see you've already lost at least a dozen pounds. You'll lose a few more during the first week, where the uterus is shrinking back to its normal size. What you have to do is be patient and give yourself time... and breast feed as much as you can. You will fit in your tight pair of jeans in a year at most. Just make sure you don't overdo sweet snacks while you breast feed. Contrary to common belief, sweets, deserts, and sugary beverages won't increase milk production, they will only make you overweight. To enhance breast milk production, drink plenty of fluids. Try and drink 2 liters of fluids a day, such as water, fresh fruit juices, milk, and herbal teas like fennel and linden. A woman who has recently given birth should definitely not follow a weight-loss diet, as she needs a lot of energy, especially if she's breastfeeding, which is a highly energy intensive activity; as the baby nurses, you will get hungry.

Taking care of a baby takes more energy than a full-time job. You will forget to even eat while looking after your child, which counts as a spontaneous kind of diet. And you can exercise by putting your baby in his stroller and going for a walk. I've never liked dieting, I wouldn't be able to stick to a diet if I wanted to anyway. I'm too fond of eating. When I'm limited as to what I can eat, it feels like the color has washed out of my life. I breastfed my son until he was two, during which time I did just the opposite of dieting, I kept snacking continuously. However, I lost weight easily thanks to spinning exercises. And it was a nice and slow weight loss, too, so it was healthy. And don't bother wearing postpartum girdles; you're wrong if you think they help shrink your belly, they just compress and immobilize the muscles. The doctors recommend exercising and following a healthy diet instead of using girdles. The recipe is simple: Drink plenty of water, take walks, and let your muscles relax!

The Miracle Of Spinning

I lost my pregnancy pounds thanks to spinning exercises. My son Matteo was seven months old and I'd introduced him to solids, therefore, I didn't have to be with him and nurse him continuously, which gave me some freedom. Most of the better gyms in Brussels have a baby care center. It's not easy to go to the gym with a baby, especially in winter time, but when you've put your mind to getting back in shape you can overcome minor difficulties like that. Besides, it's a good thing to take the baby out at least once a day, even in winter. You just have to be a little more organized to go to the gym. The preparation is tiresome, you have to pack the baby's food, his diapers, an extra set of clothes, besides your usual gym stuff, but baby care is cheaper in the gym and allows you to save time, too. If, for instance, you want to exercise for an hour, take a shower, maybe relax in the sauna for a while, get dressed and rest, you need a total of two hours. If the baby is there, you can nurse him straight away and you don't have to hurry to get home in time.

Once you've tasted adrenaline, you're addicted to it. Spinning has become one of my favorite sports along with skiing and swimming. If, like me, you have limited time and patience for gym classes, spinning is the ideal form of exercise for you. I find it to be one of the most exciting forms of gym activity. It involves riding a stationary bike to the rhythm of music, under the supervision of an instructor. It's intimidating to watch, but once you start you take to it immediately. It's great for impatient exercisers to be able to cycle in winter and summer alike, and to burn up to 500 calories in 45 minutes.

Breastfeeding

One of my twins was a boy, and the other one a girl. I had picked names for them before they were even born, the girl was Stella and the boy Teoman. Teoman was happy staying put but Stella couldn't wait to be born and to come to her mother, she ripped open her sac. They were only five months along. I had to have a premature delivery and I lost them. Meanwhile, my body was acting like that of any mother who'd just given birth and preparing to nurse. The body adjusts to breastfeeding immediately after delivery. The milk glands start working, even though you milk may not come in straight away. Normally, new mothers consume foods and drinks known to enhance breast milk production, but I had to take pills to stop it. It took time for my breasts to stop producing milk, and it felt so long to me. The same pills are used by mothers who do not wish to breastfeed, what a shame! During those hospital days where I waited for my milk to stop, I tried to figure out those mothers who chose not to breastfeed their babies, but I couldn't. And later, when I became a mother and got to breastfeed my baby, I felt they missed out on so much. Breastfeeding is a very special event in a woman's life and it's very emotional. It's an unmatched gift from the universe, a unique pleasure, it's the ultimate bonding opportunity between mother and baby. It's an experience that every mother must have if she can...[*]

---

[*] I attended a breastfeeding seminar held by WHO (the World Health Organization) in the clinic in Brussels where I delivered my son Matteo, a few weeks prior to delivery. What I learned there was extremely valuable to me. That's where I found out how important breastfeeding was for a mother and her baby. The first milk that comes in is called colostrum, it has a sweet-savory taste. It's produced during the first four or five days after delivery, for the consumption of the newborn. It contains high levels of protein and antibodies and immunoglobulin, a substance that enhances the baby's immune system. This fluid, that the breasts start to produce during the eighth month of pregnancy, is like an antibiotic that protects your baby against diseases and is irreplaceable. It's highly beneficial, even vital, for the baby to be breastfed if only for three days following delivery, if at all possible. So one should never worry about breastfeeding for too long, the longer you do it, the better it is.

The first rule in breastfeeding is to be calm and patient, and to get plenty of rest (that is, if you can) while waiting for your milk to come in. Try and stay at the hospital as long as you can and let the nurses take care of your baby for a few days, you will do it for long enough. Your milk will come in within the first few days after delivery. How soon it will be varies from woman to woman. When your breasts start producing milk, they are engorged, and the baby may have difficulty nursing properly because it's still tiny and weak, in which case the milk ducts may become clogged. A new mother may find breastfeeding difficult at first. When the baby cries hungrily, she's worried she may not be feeding it adequately and experiences stress, which is not good for her. In time, milk production becomes more regular and a bond is established between mother and child. The first month may be especially tasking but things gradually get better, and the desired outcome is achieved with a little effort and patience.

I must admit I found breastfeeding to be an ordeal at first. When I talked to a friend of mine who'd recently given birth, I saw she felt the same. We'd both always read and been told that breastfeeding was wonderful and very beneficial for mother and baby alike... until we started to do it, when we saw it could be even harder than giving birth! Nobody had told us it was going to be that painful, we were totally unprepared. They always talk about labor pain and how excruciatingly painful contractions are, but I for one experienced more pain during breastfeeding than in delivery. My milk ducts were blocked, my left breast was swollen. I remember feeling unthinkable pain, as if my nipples were being pricked by countless needles.

I can never forget one night where I cried with pain. I was in bed, with a high fever. I had a burning sensation and unbearable pain in my breast. I couldn't think of holding the baby, let alone breastfeeding. I made an effort to be sensible and do whatever needed to be done in good time; I showered my breast with cold and hot water, applied hot compresses on it, took anti-inflammatory drugs... My instinct told me this couldn't be how breastfeeding was supposed to be and that this ordeal was soon to be over. I waited patiently and endured the pain for a few months for the sake of my baby. When he was two months old, I had managed to establish a comfortable breastfeeding routine and I enjoyed it thoroughly. There was a beautiful bond between us and I was elated that I could feed him. In time, I became an expert in it, I could breastfeed anywhere I went, which made life so much easier. It was extremely convenient as breast milk always came in the right temperature and ready to use, it didn't require warming or sterilizing, so I needed nothing else but a scarf to cover my feeding baby. I could watch with teary eyes in admiration as he nursed.

The Benefits Of Breastfeeding

Breastfeeding is in again! Celebrities' babies who used to grow up on the bottle lest their mothers end up with sagging breasts and dark circles around the eyes are rejoined with their mother's bosom once more. Breastfeeding is the new trend worldwide. Experts emphasize that it's beneficial both for mother and baby. First of all, it decreases the mother's risk of breast cancer. Furthermore, it allows you to lose weight and to bond with your baby, and it's good for the psychological health of both.

•   Breast milk protects the baby against diseases. Diarrhea, allergies, respiratory tract infections, asthma, diabetes, obesity, and coronary heart disease are seen less commonly in breastfed babies. Breast milk enhances the baby's immune system. Nursing is good for its oral and dental health. And close contact during nursing helps mental and physical development. Breast milk contains the growth factor enhancing and regulating the growth of all organs and systems. Another amazing fact about breast milk is that its composition is not fixed but changes with time to parallel the baby's physiological development. For instance, the milk that you produce during the first month is not suitable for your baby's needs at three months. So don't keep the milk that you express in the freezer any longer than you have to. Every mother produces just the right milk for her baby's needs. For all these reasons, no formula can possibly replace breast milk. A baby must be breastfed exclusively for the first six months if possible.

•   When you breastfeed you don't need to follow a diet because you will be shedding pounds automatically. While I was breastfeeding, I ate more than ever, I ate whatever I felt like and even what I didn't feel like, yet I saw I'd lost a few more pounds when I stepped on the scale every week. It was awesome! To eat her way to a slimmer body is every woman's dream, and breastfeeding makes it come true. Your weight keeps going up while you're pregnant and down while you're breastfeeding. It may look like a sedentary activity but a woman who breastfeeds seven or eight times a day burns an extra 400 to 500 calories, comparable to daily exercise, and at the end of the day you really feel as if you've been exercising. Breastfeeding absorbs all your energy, until you feel you cannot lift a finger. It's a natural diet program!

• Breastfeeding establishes mental connection between mother and child. The baby has psychological needs that must be met from the moment where it's born, the need for safety is one of those. It wants to be held by its mother, to feel her scent and her warmth. Likewise, the mother's hormones work better if she's close to her baby and can feel his smell. The experts even recommend that the mother and the baby sleep in the same room, at least during the first months, as it enhances milk production and keeps the baby calmer and more peaceful. Sometimes the baby cannot nurse and the mother has to express breast milk and feed it to the baby in a bottle. This could never compare to the baby's nursing directly from the mother's breast. You shouldn't use a bottle unless you have to. If the baby gets used to the bottle, it will breastfeed less and less every day and milk supply will dwindle. While I lived in Spain, I saw mothers who chose not to breastfeed even though they did have breast milk. It might be liberating to have the option not to breastfeed but it causes the baby and the mother to miss out on those special moments. During the 22 months I breastfed my son, I sometimes complained, or felt exhausted, but I chose to insist on breastfeeding and I'm very happy to have experienced this unique feeling...

And The Downside

Breastfeeding may become a nightmare in spite of all the benefits mentioned above:

• A woman must be careful with what she eats or drinks while breastfeeding. You may feel as if you were on a never ending diet starting with pregnancy in the first place. Although it's not like a weight-loss diet, it's still limiting. Most vegetables might cause flatulence in the baby. You're not supposed to eat any beans and it's hard to go through winter without eating any beans, chick peas, or lentils. Let's say you just decided to ignore the warning and had some, then you have to stay up all night trying to soothe your baby writhing in gas pain, and you pay dearly for your meal. You cannot drink alcohol, as it gets into your breast milk. To think every bite and every gulp that goes in your mouth will go to the baby may became tiresome after a while.

• Breastfeeding increases the baby's dependence on you, making you an inseparable couple. Who wants to be separated from her baby anyway? But sometimes you feel like taking a holiday alone with your husband, or to have an undisturbed night's sleep. The babies will feed on breast milk (or formula) for the first six months, and solids are introduced only after the fifth or sixth month, the doctors differ as to their opinion about the point at which solids can or should be introduced, it may also vary from country to country. If you're breastfeeding, you have to be there to feed your baby every two to three hours, unless you can clone yourself or have a wet nurse to replace you. There may be places where you have to be and cannot take your baby, in which case you have to time your errand very carefully. You have to leave immediately after you've fed your baby and come back in three hours. It's an idea to express milk and let someone else give it to the baby, but experts warn about bottle feeding newborns, as they may find it easier and refuse the breast afterwards. As I was afraid of this, I didn't give my baby the bottle during the first four months. But he became addicted to the breast and he refused the bottle, he frowned and turned his face away, as if saying he wouldn't think of nursing on a piece of plastic instead of my soft, warm, pillow-like breasts where he could rest his head. All my attempts failed and Matteo grew up without ever nursing on a bottle or a pacifier. It was hard for me at times but I left it up to him, because I could. I didn't really insist, because I had only him to take care of then, so I had enough time and energy. But I introduced my younger son Leo to the bottle earlier on and he enjoyed both the breast and the bottle equally.

My Son Is Addicted To The Breast!

Matteo took so much pleasure in nursing that I couldn't bring myself to take it away from him and I didn't wean him until he was almost two. That's why he's never forgotten about the breast, he knows it very well and gazes at it admiringly, no matter whose breast it is.

Matteo loved the newborn puppies of our neighbor, he went to see them every day. He picked up the puppies, talked to them, and when the mother came he affectionately put them to her breast, and encouraged them to nurse. Once I told him that babies need to nurse a lot to grow up, he never forgot this, and as he saw my bulging belly he kept telling me that he wanted to hold his little brother when he would be born and feed him. Sometimes he would put his ear to my belly and listened quietly. When I asked him what the baby said, he answered: "He says 'brother'!" When he saw me changing clothes, he tried to nurse on my breasts. When I told him that his little brother would need them when he would be born, he said he could let his brother have one and keep one for himself. But when his brother was born, contrary to my expectations, he didn't try to join him in nursing, he just expressed he wasn't pleased about my sharing a special moment with his baby brother by pulling at my clothes and complaining about my not playing with him.

Is Breastfeeding In Public Regarded As Inappropriate In Turkey?

Breastfeeding in public is perceived as the most natural thing on earth in foreign countries while it can be regarded as inappropriate in Turkey. Matteo was born in Brussels and he spent the first couple of years of his life there. We were out together all the time and feeding him in public was nothing but natural to me and to the people around. But Leo was born in Turkey and we stayed there until he was 7 weeks old. I was sitting on a bench in a mall, breastfeeding him when a security guard approached me and warned me that I had quite an audience. When I looked up, I couldn't believe my eyes as I saw there was a group of men staring at me from the gallery of the upper floor. In Turkey, you'll find many sick men who perceive breastfeeding in public as exhibition issue and feel it's alright to stare at your breasts when you're feeding your child. Newborn babies need to feed every two to three hours. If you decide to nurse them only when you're at home, it would be impossible for you to go out. For your own comfort, ask the people in charge to show you to a private area suitable for nursing. In some malls and larger shops they have nursing rooms. If there isn't one, use the changing room in a clothes shop, no one will dare kick out a nursing baby. In a pinch, you could always nurse in your car. There is always a way of avoiding prying eyes.

Motherhood = Sleepness Nights

Sleeplessness will start before the baby is even born, during pregnancy. Some will suffer from loss of sleep due to morning sickness during the first trimester. In later stages of pregnancy, with the pressure of the growing uterus on the bladder, frequent bathroom trips may be necessary. I'd recommend you to limit your fluid intake before going to bed. The sweetest phase of sleep is the REM phase, which comes just before sun rise... If you're expecting your first baby, you're lucky, you can always stay in bed till late even if you haven't been able to get enough sleep at night. The smartest thing to do during this period is to accept all offers to help, which allows you to save all your energy for your baby and to please your family and friends at the same time. To grow a baby in your belly is a tiring job, you have to get plenty of rest. Try and get some shut eye during the day. It's almost impossible to have an uninterrupted night's sleep during pregnancy, if you are among those who can, consider yourself lucky, of all the pregnant women I've known, I've not come across one who could sleep throughout the night, for several reasons. Your large belly makes it hard to find a comfortable sleeping position and the fluctuations in your body temperature disturb you in your sleep, you will wake up hot and sweaty in the middle of the night. It's as if your body were turned into a factory operating non-stop 24 hours a day, sleep eludes you.

Still, you are entitled to sleep and rest as much as you want (that is, if you can) while you're expecting, but once the expected guest has arrived the situation will be changed. I don't like sleeping during the day. I dislike lying down lazily when it's light outside. I feel napping is a waste of time, especially in summer, when the sun is shining bright and everybody is out in the street. Don't we waste enough time sleeping through the night? I prefer to sleep at night, and 6 to 7 hours of sleep is more than enough for me. Once I see the morning light, I cannot sleep any longer. Even on weekends, when I stay at home, I don't sleep during the day, I just lie around lazily, wrap myself up in my blanket, get lost in dreams, think about things to do, engage in small talk with my sweetheart or have a conversation about nice things. But then, all these are pleasures of the past, belonging to our days B.C. – before the child! I always heard that having a child would change my lifestyle, but I never understood how much before I experienced it firsthand. When I was expecting my older son, I was supposed to stay in bed until term and all my friends with children told me it was a great opportunity for me to get plenty of rest and sleep. "You'll never get the chance again," they said, "sleep all you can before the baby arrives." Now I know that I should have stocked up on sleep! When you've spent six months with a newborn baby, it's painful to look back on the days where you had the opportunity to sleep and didn't use it. When you're exhausted of feeding and burping the baby throughout the night, you feel you could give up so much just to get a little sleep, whether at daytime or at nighttime! You don't care whether the sun's shining outside anymore, all you want is to close your eyes and sleep...

Fathers Can Take Care Of Babies, Too

What do women look for in a man? What do they expect from men? Of course, the first thing you expect is to share your life with your partner, other than that, if you're not married you want to share your social life, if you're newly married you want them to do their share of the housework, and if you have a newborn baby, you want them to share the baby's care. And they have to do their share without your having to ask them. It's always all about sharing. While women are born programmed to share, for men it's a skill that needs to be learned. I admire the new generation of men. The modern living conditions and the handy, innovative baby products facilitate baby care for men, so that dads can now go further than just loving their children and take active part in bringing them up. This allows moms to go back to work, socialize, and make more time for themselves, which in turn makes them feel more at peace with themselves, a feeling that reflects on the whole family. It's very common in Europe, especially northern Europe, for dads to take a stroll with their babies in the park, to feed them, while moms are at the beauty parlor having a facial, at the mall shopping, or at a café catching up with friends, even though it would still be a rare sight in Turkey. Once, newborn babies would always be on the mother's lap or back, but now we can see many fathers feeding, burping, and changing their babies. This new model of behavior contradicts the old way of categorizing chores as men's jobs and women's jobs, men can very well take care of babies. For instance, my husband was very good at lulling our son to sleep. Matteo wasn't a baby who liked to sleep, it took a long time to put him to bed and I found it tiring. But Cosimo had a special gift; I still don't know how exactly he did it but he could quickly convince Matteo to go to bed. He would tell or read him stories, and then tell him to go to bed, and Matteo would do as he was told, close his eyes and go to sleep.

A Call To Fathers-To-Be

New dads, or dads-to-be, please make a point of reading parenting/ child rearing books with your spouse and getting ready to take care of your baby together. Some of the things you read in books will turn out to be somewhat different in real life, but it's still good to be prepared. Don't assume you won't be needed because your wife will be there, all prepared and well equipped for the job. You'll see there will be a lot for you to do and you'll enjoy doing it, too. After all, there's no law saying that it's up to the mother to do everything about the baby. Fathers can easily give their baby a bottle, bathe him, burp him, put him to bed or change him. Although they cannot breastfeed, they can always help the mother while she does. Nursing a baby is exhausting and dehydrating, so you could wait on your nursing wife. You could bring her a drink, or cook for her while she's breastfeeding.

My husband has always helped me much in caring for our children. He's a doting, caring father. Sometimes he even takes it too far and makes us laugh. He's always been fussy, but he seems to have gotten fussier since he became a father. Here's a funny story which still makes me laugh as I recall it. Cosimo would often come home during his lunch break as he missed our son and wanted to see him. It was one of those days, he'd just popped in to give

Matteo a hug although he was rather short on time, he was to go to an important meeting at the European Parliament, and he was dressed up very elegantly, he had his best suit on, with a crisp white shirt, stylish cufflinks, and a grey silk tie. He picked up Matteo, a month old then, as he always did, kissed him, and then pressed his lips on the baby's brow. Next, he turned to me and said: "I think he's got a fever." I was used to hearing this line, at the beginning I used to take it seriously, get the thermometer and take the baby's fever, but as it turned out to be a false alarm every time, I'd learnt to say: "Would you like to get the thermometer and check?" So, that's what I said, and Cosimo got the thermometer, laid our son on the changing table, unfastened his diaper and inserted the tip of the thermometer into his rectum. As chance would have it, our son was ready to go... the touch of the thermometer speeded things up, so that he almost exploded, and my husband found himself on the trajectory of a projectile poop shower! As we both screamed, my mother and our helper Mrs. Gülten came running in the nursery, and doubled up in laughter when they saw this hilarious scene. Cosimo started laughing, too, after he got over the first shock. His suit was ruined, but Matteo looked just fine, not feverish at all. My husband never touched the thermometer again after that day!

Being An Expat = Moving Often

I first heard the word 'expat' when I actually became one myself. It's used to designate a person who moves from one county to another for work... Expats share the same destiny as diplomats, so they understand each other very well and become good friends when they meet. If you wonder what it's like to be an expat, it's living with the constant sensation of driving a brand new car. On one hand, it's new and exciting, on the other, it's stressful and tiresome...

The prospect of living and working abroad seems appealing, and it really is. Most of us dream of living in a different country, getting to know the people, being one of them... I've been living as an expat for years and I've enjoyed it tremendously, but before you start to enjoy it there is a difficult transition period. You have to strive and struggle go get anything. First of all, you have to have a suitable personality; you have to be flexible, adaptable, and sociable, you have to be able to communicate easily, you have to like change, and novelty as well as struggle. You have to be willing to learn the language, and have the talent to learn it. It's not for you if you're one of those who miss your country's food and TV shows, your family and friends back there as soon as you've been away for three days. It's definitely not for you if you're a creature of habit, you may never be happy as an expat. I've moved five times and stayed in countless hotels in four different countries during the last seven years. We're about to move again for the sixth time. We've never been able to finish unpacking for good for 10 years. Every house requires you to get new things for various reasons, and you have a hard time finding a place for everything in your next house. We're a couple who doesn't like to live in a place like it was a temporary arrangement, we like to settle properly. Every house is different and calls for different pieces of furniture, and we can never feel comfortable until we've got everything we need to make a new house completely ours. We have that bookcase, designed by Rod Arad, which takes three people and six hours to install; it's just a shelf for books, but it's a strange piece that you have to manually put into shape. Every time we move, we take our time and install it in the best corner of the living room, and place hundreds of books and magazines on it one by one, leafing through them, sometimes sitting down to read them, and throwing away some of them.

We spend so much time and energy each time we move house that we promise ourselves and each other that next time we won't establish ourselves so thoroughly, but we soon forget our promises, we're incurable. When you're an architect and your husband is crazy about decoration, you can't help it, you have to make a house yours even if you know you'll live there only for a year. I move the furniture around in the hotel rooms where I'll only be staying for a night, let alone a place where I'll spend a few years! Moving and going to another country is exciting when you're a childless couple. Walking the streets to find a house is the best way to get to know a city. You learn the language, familiarize yourself with the culture, you see a lot of places, you don't live like a tourist but like a native, you adapt to the lifestyle, and you learn from it as well as enjoy it tremendously. When you 'go native,' that is, when you adopt the lifestyle of the country, you get to meet the local people. You start getting acquainted with your neighbors, your mailman, the baker on your street, your spouse's co-workers, the people who go to the same gym as you, and you get over the feeling of loneliness. Besides, your life standard and earning level is higher as an expat than in your own country, the company often pays the rent, so you get to live in a nice house in an upscale neighborhood.

Moving Must Be Part Of My Destiny

They say a change is as good as resting, which is definitely true for me. It's nice and refreshing to make a change, and it's a new life experience, it's an opportunity not to be missed. A new start is difficult but exciting and reviving. If you miss your old routine, too bad for you, because a new house means a new life and new habits. But you have to see it as fun. Just imagine, your company gives you rather a generous allowance for rent so you can pick any house you fancy. It's nice to collect objects that belong to the countries you go to, to keep them in showcases, and to look at them to recall the good old days you spent there. And you'll make friends from all over the world, who'll introduce you to the traditional dishes, customs, and lifestyles of their countries, expanding your horizon. Your children will learn two or more languages simultaneously.

Basically, everything unfolds as you hoped. These are the good things about being an expat. But the other side of the coin is to wake up from the dream once all the firsts have been experienced and the excitement of novelty wears off, to have to face the reality of where you live and to find you don't like it, which is also quite common in an expat's life. Man likes the feeling of belonging somewhere, he finds it comforting and reassuring. I've known people who live in hotels throughout their lives, most of them are either single, or children of mixed-nationality families, or they have no other choice because of the nature of their job.

I must say, though, that it is unusual to see a person who still lives with their family after getting married and having children, of course, there can be exceptions. I met a family with two children who were in Istanbul for a while and they lived in the Hilton. They were an interesting, crazy family, the most easygoing and careless people I've ever known. I must admit there have been moments in my life where I had difficulties, even though I have a very flexible personality and adapt easily to all kinds of environments. You have to start from scratch every time, you have to find a new house, settle in, meet people, find schools for your children if you have any, help them settle in their new schools, arrange social activities for your children and yourself, apply for legal permits, complete the required legal documentation for work, health care and residence, find a doctor for your family, and very often, as you are busy with all this, you neglect your own career and it falls to the bottom of your list of priorities.

If you wish to work, you have to learn the language really well, which means you first have to go back to being a student and enroll in a language class. The new language will confuse you, you try to put what you've learned in the language class to use, you struggle to communicate with the people in the shops and in the streets, and you cannot express yourself adequately, and come home with a terrible headache. The dictionary becomes a permanent resident of your purse. When you need medication, you have to use the dictionary and your inadequate language skills to communicate with the pharmacist, telling the doctor what's ailing you is an ordeal.

It's almost impossible to pursue your career, to practice your profession as an expat wife. Very often, you face accreditation problems, that is, your diploma is not accepted as valid in the new country. Especially if you're a Turkish citizen, you're in trouble, it makes everything twice as hard! But if you have an independent, 'moveable' job, if you're for instance a painter or a writer or have a job that you can practice online, then it would make your life much easier.

You might think of building yourself a new career, but it depends on how long you intend to stay in that country. If you plan to stay only a short while, then it's not worth the effort. Following your husband as an expat wife means you have to make sacrifices concerning your career. You'll always be the one hunting for a job because your husband will have his position waiting for him, the only change he has to deal with is his new working environment, new co-workers, and maybe new responsibilities, while you will not have a job, not even a working permit in the new country. Some companies will even prohibit the spouses from working.

Even if you aren't allowed to work, it's hard to find a job where you can pursue a career. The jobs that you're most likely to get are temporary or short-contract positions, even if you decide to take them, they will not further your career so you'll look the more unsuccessful and the more useless for it and experience a personal failure in your career. If you don't work, you'll be regarded as an expat wife who's dependent on her husband, who prefers to live comfortably instead of working, maybe even as lazy, and you'll blame yourself. You become a housewife even if you had a good job back in your country. Sometimes, this temporary situation may work for you. Your work life may have bored or wore you down, you may want to take a break and devote more time to yourself and your family.

It's a great opportunity to plan to have children. You can spend as much time as you wish with your child and enjoy parenting. Then have another one straight away or after waiting a while till your first child gets a little older, expand your family, when your youngest one reaches the age of three, put them into daycare and take up your career where you've left off. Or you can go back to college or university to continue your education, maybe even study a new subject that you find exciting, take up a new profession or hobby. How enticing is that?

Sometimes, however, you find you cannot keep this optimistic attitude in the face of things. It hurts you to have to start from scratch and to be regarded as 'unqualified' when you had a good job and earned your living back in your country. You may have to be the party who makes sacrifices because of your husband's position. It's your choice and there's no one to blame, but it can still make you feel anxious, hopeless, and weary, it can go as far as hurting your marriage. Therefore you should weigh the pros and cons of your decision carefully at the beginning. A healthy, happy mother means healthy, happy children. The adults will be the ones most affected by the decision to be an expat, children are quicker to adapt to new circumstances.

"I don't play tennis with angry expat women who feel entrapped," says Robin Pascoe, a Canadian woman who's changed four countries in 15 years, "they hit the ball with all their anger. There are two kinds of expat wives; those who are happy with the change and those who are not. The ones that are unhappy will call their husbands like 20 times a day, both husbands and wives are desperate." Robin has followed her husband to several countries because of his job, and she has managed to transform her lifestyle and her experiences. She's written five books about expat life, where she tells about the difficulties she's had, hoping to help those who take the same path. She defines herself as an 'expat expert' and is a world-renowned author. She's enjoyed so much attention that she's started to write columns in international newspapers.

When you move to a country of which you're unfamiliar with the language, the people, the habits and customs, the geography, the towns, the countryside, you feel like a fish out of the water for a while, until you settle. It's not easy to build a new life in a new country. International companies that have workers relocate overseas every few years should offer orientation programs for the families. I've often wondered how the companies that are so businesslike can ignore this issue.

I relocated three times to follow my husband who was appointed to another country and had to suspend my career as an architect for a while. While I focused on building a family during this time, I tried to keep abreast of the developments and trends in my profession. When we first moved to Barcelona, I joined the 'International Women Network', following the advice of friends I'd made there. At the end of the first meeting I went to, the new members were supposed to go on stage and make a brief speech to introduce themselves. When it was my turn, I told I was an architect and I'd come to Barcelona from Istanbul.

At the end of the meeting, I was surrounded by women who wanted to talk with me, they must have found it interesting that I was a Turkish architect. Their attention pleased me much and I took to the club at once. Nice, stylish, lively ladies were asking me to help them decorate their houses; I was lucky, I'd found myself a job without even having to seek it. I was commissioned some projects in Barcelona thanks to the club. These expat wives who had come to spend a few years in Barcelona because of their husbands' work lived in leased houses that didn't feel like home.

They wanted to decorate their houses to suit their needs and tastes but weren't willing to invest too much on the decoration of a house where they weren't be staying but a few years.

I could understand it only too well as I experienced the same thing. It's hard to live in a house that feels like a hotel room even for a few years. As the men are at work all day, it's up to us women to make the houses livable, to transform them to suit our lifestyles. My first clients were Pamela from Poland and Nicole from the U.S., with whom I later became close friends. Pamela needed a play room in her house for her two sons. And the overall ambiance of the house was a bit sad. The furniture consisted of odd pieces which lacked harmony and made the house look untidy. The house needed order, color, taste and ambiance. We achieved a new look with a fresh wall paint, new floors in some of the rooms, new curtains and carpets, a bookcase, toy cases for the children's room, lighting fixtures, and some accessories, without having to make drastic changes. Pamela was pleased with the result. I got her beautiful couch and bed covers and pillow cases from the Covered Bazaar in Istanbul, and we bought the remaining items from other shops like Ikea and Habitat. Pamela was happy that we achieved such a nice change on a reasonable budget and she felt much better about her house that she found tastelessly decorated earlier. And I was pleased with the job I'd done, besides, I'd learnt a great deal while working on a project in a strange country.

During the period where I lived in Barcelona, I worked as a business agent for Derin Design in Spain as well as undertaking some interior design projects involving homes or cafés. Derin Design the famous brand of furniture by Aziz Sarıyer, one of Turkey's prominent designers. I managed to sell Derin's items to furniture shops where they'd never heard of the brand before or were even surprised that the Turkish designed furniture. This gave me the opportunity to meet many people and to advance my level of Spanish very fast thanks to extensive practice during the interviews. I congratulated myself for bravely introducing the brand to the purchasing agents in architects' offices and furniture shops in spite of my inarticulate Spanish.

It's not easy to do business in Barcelona and in Catalonia. A tourist wouldn't notice it, but the Catalans are not very open to novelty and strangers and tend to favor their countrymen, it takes time to convince them to embrace something new. But at the end of the second year, there were practically no furniture shop left in Catalonia unfamiliar with Derin. Just as business was starting to improve, we moved to Brussels. I had to discontinue my activities as Derin Design already had an agent in Belgium. Despite all the difficulties it entailed, living in different countries brought depth to my soul if not to my pockets. Barcelona inspired me, contributed to my professional qualities, my taste and culture with its architectural and aesthetic riches. Brussels allowed me to have two healthy sons, although after much struggle. And Italy will be where I take up my career and business life after a long break and where the pieces of my life fall into place to complete the mosaic.

Acknowledgements

Life is beautiful despite all its difficulties. It's a combination of dreams and reality, a blend of sweet and bitter tastes, an intersection of people's paths... Sometimes dreams come true in real life. And when they do, you forget all the pains of the past, especially when this dream come true is a new life that comes into the world, a gift that's bestowed upon you, the fruit of your love...

While writing this book, that I dedicate to my sons Matteo and Leo, and to my babies that I've lost, I found myself sometimes teary eyed with a lump in my throat, and sometimes with a smile on my face. The idea of writing a book first came about when I lost my twins at the fifth month of my pregnancy. I thought I had to put to words what I'd been through, so other women who tread the same path would know they're not alone. During that period, many times I started to write but couldn't go on as I burst into tears. There was more than just pain to what I'd been through, there was much more I wanted to tell, but apparently I wasn't ready to tell my story yet.

I deferred my project but it went on by itself, as I spent time with my woman friends and listened to their stories, which would bring depth to my book. I put their stories next to mine and I put pen to paper once more when I felt I was ready for it, unaware of the new life that was starting in me. As chance would have it, the conception of my baby coincided with my beginning to write this book, which was going to become more colorful with the introduction of my second baby into my life.

Life is full of surprises. Only a few years ago I was desperate to have a baby, and here I am now, with two. I consider myself among the luckiest women on earth, like all the women who have babies or who have become mothers otherwise. So, thank you, God. Thank you, nature...

Thank you my sons, my dearest Matteo and Leo, a thousand times, for letting me enjoy motherhood and feel this love...

Thank you, my romantic husband, my love, my mentor, my friend, my partner, my everything, for making me feel special and always being there for me, and for being a great father...

Dad! My darling father, thank you for bringing me up strong, for supporting me in every way throughout my life, and for always being ready to give me an encouraging, heartening talk even though we may be miles apart...

Thank you, my one and only brother Can, for letting me experience sisterly love, a feeling so similar to motherhood, when you were born, for being my brother, and for still allowing me to act as your big sister...

And mom! My dearest mother... You always said, "You'll see when you have children!" You were right! I now understand you so much better, being a mother myself. Thank you for giving me life, for raising me as a good person, for rallying around me whenever I needed you, no matter what the circumstances, for loving me with an unfailing love, without ever expecting anything in return, for undertaking a job as tough as motherhood and bringing me up to this day...

I would also like to thank my American publishing house, St. Michael's press, who gave me the courage and endless support to publish this book in English.

THANK YOU ALL ENDLESSLY...

www.ingramcontent.com/pod-product-compliance
Lightning Source LLC
LaVergne TN
LVHW091212080426
835509LV00009B/957